The Essential Carer's Guide

Second edition

Mary Jordan

First published in 2013 by Hammersmith Health Books – an imprint of
Hammersmith Books Limited
14 Greville Street, London EC1N 8SB, UK
www.hammersmithbooks.co.uk

British Library Cataloguing in Publication Data: A CIP record of this
book is available from the British Library.

ISBN (print edition): 978-1-78161-025-1
ISBN (ebook): 978-1-78161-026-8

Commissioning editor: Georgina Bentliff
Designed and typeset by: Julie Bennett
Proof reading: Helen Clutton
Index: Dr Laurence Errington
Production: Helen Whitehorn, Pathprojects
Printed and bound by TJ International Limited

Contents

About the Author

Mary Jordan has extensive experience of both sides of caring, as a carer to friends and relatives and, more recently, professionally through her work with a national dementia charity where she daily supports people with a diagnosis of dementia and their carers. For many years she worked for the National Health Service and has served in the Armed Forces. In addition to articles and papers published in medical, nursing and social care journals and general magazines, Mary is also known for her books *The Essential Guide to Avoiding Dementia: understanding the risks*, *The Fundholder's Handbook* and the award-winning *End of Life: the Essential Guide to Caring*.

Acknowledgements

Although I have written from the starting point of my own experience, I have had to do considerable research and I have been helped by many people. In writing the first edition, I was particularly helped by, and would like to thank again: Professor Basant Puri MA(Cantab), PhD, MB BChir, BSc(Hons) MathSci, MRPSych, DipStat, MMath for his advice on the previous Mental Health Act and his valuable comments on Nutrition for the elderly; Dr Helen McGinty MB ChB, MRCGP, for editing the chapter on medical matters; Sharon Boylett MSc, PGDip, NDN, DipN, RGN, for the information she gave about the service provided by district nurses; Seamus Mahon for advice on nursing and care homes; and Mick Hanneghan for information about social services. For developing the second edition I would particularly like to thank Frances Leckie of Independent Living for her help and advice on areas where revision and greater detail were needed.

The case histories in this book have come from many sources and, as before, I wish to thank Patricia Palmer, Peter Palmer, Sara Clayton, Joan Zilva and Liz Jones specifically. Some who have passed on their own experiences have asked to remain anonymous but I give them my thanks for their contributions.

For the photographs in chapters 1 and 3, I would like to thank: the Ability Superstore (for Figures 1 to 5), Pivotell Ltd (for their advance pill dispenser – Figure 6), and Stannah (for their Active Rollator – Figure 7).

Acknowledgements

I would not have been able to complete the first edition of this book without the support of my husband, Chris, and the rest of my family. For this second edition I must particularly thank my son, Tristram, and daughter-in-law Erica Arnold for their help.

Preface

I am pleased to be able to offer a second edition of my guide for carers. The idea for the first edition came from my personal experience of acting as a carer, and I have updated the original version in response to the very welcome feedback I have received from readers. As a carer, once I started talking about my experiences and the problems I was encountering I began to realise that there were many, many carers out there. Everyone who is a carer wants to do their best for the one they are caring for and everyone seems to have a story to tell about their experiences. I received a lot of support from others in my period as a carer and exchanged much helpful information. I thought it would be useful if the information I collected and the experience I gained could be pulled together in one place, but it also seemed to me that a book like this could be more than a collection of facts. So I have included case stories wherever I have thought them relevant.

As with the first edition, all the stories in this book are true stories, although sometimes the relationships have been changed to protect identities. In this way I hope that, in reading this book, you will gain something of the experience of belonging to a support group – in other words, the feeling that you are not alone and that you can gain from reading someone else's solutions to similar problems. Support groups are something I would recommend. It is really good to know that you are not alone, and often others have encountered the same problem as you are experiencing and are able to give you tips to manage the situation. Today there are also many online forums available which act in the same way as support groups so that, even if you find it very hard to leave the house to attend a group, you can access this kind of 'virtual' support.

I also wanted to make this book a resource tool – a start on the research path to finding help and support. So I have included 'Further useful information' at the end of the book. All contact details have been checked and updated for the second edition, with many new websites added, which can be directly linked from the ebook edition.

For this second edition I have changed the way the book is organised, partly on the advice of readers of the first edition. You can still use the book as a resource tool to look for information about just one area of caring; alternatively, you may want to learn about the whole subject and read the book from beginning to end. If you do so, you will inevitably find some repetition, but I hope this makes the book more helpful rather than otherwise.

Much of the information in this book will be relevant to you if you are caring for a younger person, whether a relative or not, but the emphasis is on the increasing physical and mental frailty of old age.

There is an enormous amount of information here, yet I know it is not comprehensive. If there is something important you think should be added, please write to me c/o Hammersmith Health Books (info@hammersmithbooks.co.uk) or contact me via my website: www.maryjordan.co.uk

Chapter 1

First steps – occupational therapy assessment, aids and equipment

My parents-in-law had seemed completely self-sufficient. I had noticed that he seemed to be getting rather autocratic with her but just put this down to 'old age crankiness'. Then he was taken ill with pneumonia and we all realised suddenly that she was quite incapable of looking after him properly. He had been compensating for her memory lapses and loss of ability by giving her direct instruction all through the day. ('Get up now, Freda,' 'Get ready to go shopping now,' 'Give me your washing to put in the machine.') We honestly had no idea until then that she was suffering from the beginnings of dementia.

****

Sometimes we see at an early stage that elderly relatives or friends need a little help. In some cases they will voluntarily ask for help, but very often they will not, seeing it as a weakness (a sign of growing old!) or as an imposition on younger family or friends to ask of their time. It can be a small thing that makes us aware – noticing difficulty with carrying shopping, for example, or realising that someone is reluctant to leave the house or to pay visits. Very often an elderly couple will become used to compensating for weakness in each other. The wife will start driving the car when her husband has been the main driver up until then, because he says one day that he is too tired. In reality perhaps he realises that his vision is not as good as it was. Or perhaps the husband starts to do the supermarket shop because his wife begins to forget essential items. Unless they are very close and visiting every day, these small adjustments may go unnoticed by friends and family until a crisis happens. Frequently, the sudden illness, admission to hospital or death of one partner brings a shocked realisation to the relatives, friends or neighbours and 'crisis management' has to be resorted to. Family and friends may not be aware that there is help available, or they may find that the elderly person continually refuses to accept 'charity'. There is often a horror of 'free' help or anything that smacks of 'social security'. Frail people about to be discharged from hospital may refuse all help, insisting that their family can 'do all that is needed'.

****

We knew Mum and Dad were getting more frail but they seemed able to manage on a day-to-day basis and one or other of us was always around at the weekend. But one weekday I finished work early and dropped in. The house was freezing cold. The fire which ran the central heating via a back boiler had gone out. It was tricky to light and Dad had always been in charge of the job. But on this day he had put his back out and was unable to get out of his chair. I found Mum in tears trying desperately to light the fire under his increasingly irate instructions. She had arthritic hands and couldn't manage. This incident made the whole family think more carefully about how they could help.

****

It is very worthwhile at this stage to get together and agree co-operation as a family, or as a group of friends. Lack of co-operation may turn out to be the biggest underlying problem as time goes on. Resentment and hostility quickly build up in the absence of communication. Guilt plays a part. A daughter living some distance away may really resent the 'hands-on' care given by a daughter-in-law even whilst knowing and understanding that she is unable to give it herself. A son may not feel at all able to give this kind of care and may react by belittling the care given by his sisters. Group meetings early on, where concrete plans can be made and (if possible) where recriminations are withheld, will help avoid such situations developing. If someone lives too far away to help with daily care, perhaps they can agree to come and stay at intervals and give 'holiday cover' to the chief carer. Someone who is not good at practical personal care may instead be able to manage the financial affairs. It helps to make use of personal strengths here. Someone who enjoys cooking may agree to keep the freezer stocked with ready meals whilst someone who is only free once a week but is a car driver might organise the shopping. A family member who works within the health service may act as the co-ordinator for healthcare.

If you appear to be the only person available to help with care, you should not try to take on everything alone. There may well be neighbours or friends of the person you are caring for who will help in the same way that family might do. Otherwise you will have to turn to professional help. Indeed, some elderly people prefer the notion that any help they are receiving is 'paid' help and not done as a favour.

Available help

There are a vast number of practical things that can be done to help those you care for live independently for longer. Occasionally, elderly people who are aware of their increasing difficulties will arrange help for themselves. Otherwise it may fall to the carer to do this. The following information is meant as a guide to what is available.

Occupational therapists

The services of an occupational therapist are usually available free of charge and you can gain access to their help through your local council, your GP or community nursing service, or through social services. Occupational therapists (OTs) are trained to assess the ability to manage everyday tasks and to give advice on selecting aids and appliances or making adaptations to the home environment which might help. You can ask for an OT assessment for the person you are caring for. If she or he has spent some time in hospital (following a stroke or a fall, for example) then s/he is unlikely to be discharged until an OT assessment has been carried out. Most community hospitals have units where they can check on the ability of patients due for discharge to carry out simple tasks (such as making a cup of tea), but if the person you care for has been in hospital for some time, and particularly if s/he lives alone, the OT team will probably take her/him home for a visit of a couple of hours, during which time they will carry out the assessment. If you can arrange it, then it is worth being present at the assessment so that you can bring up any concerns you have.

A thorough assessment will include a check of the home surroundings and in his/her report the OT will note if such items as ramps or grab-handles need to be provided and point out potential hazards such as loose rugs or trailing cables, as well as guiding the person you are caring for through some everyday tasks and recommending aids and equipment which might be helpful. OTs are especially helpful if major items like stair-lifts or wheelchairs need purchasing.

It is important that you ask to see a copy of the OT assessment report. It has happened that the report has been sent directly to the GP and is never seen by the family. It will be dutifully filed on your cared-for's notes and you may never gain the full information you need.

If you cannot get OT advice quickly by any of the routes listed above, then you might consider using a private OT service, but for this you will, of course, have to pay.

Your relative or friend may be upset, or even hostile to the OT assessment, thinking that it is aimed at proving that s/he cannot manage and will have to 'go into a home'. The very opposite is true and you should try to reassure her/him. For some years there has been a big move towards 'care in the community' and the OT team will be trying to provide all possible help to ensure that the person you are caring for can manage at home for as long as possible.

Basic help to make everyday life easier

Even without an OT assessment or purchasing any aids, you as the carer can make sure that home is safer and more convenient for the person you are caring for. Lighting is very important. Replace lightbulbs promptly and use the highest wattage which the light shade and fitting allow. Consider free- standing or wall-mounted spotlights near to chairs used for reading, knitting etc. Make sure that stair lights can be switched on and off both at the top and at the bottom of the stairs and that halls and passageways are very well lit. A light-coloured paint or paper on the walls helps to make the most of the light. Kitchens may need extra 'spot' lighting around food preparation areas and bathrooms near mirrors.

Stairs and hallways need to be kept clear of clutter as much as possible and, again, pale floor coverings help to make obstacles more visible. A second handrail can be fitted to most staircases if required (on the wall side). Small rugs should either be taken up or backed with non-slip matting or backing. Loose edges to carpets should be fixed firmly down.

Grab rails can be fitted quite easily by someone reasonably competent in DIY. These can be bought using specialist mail order catalogues or ordered online and are very useful in the bathroom and around front and back entrances, especially if there are any steps to be negotiated.

If you look around the house with the person you are caring for, you may both agree on some simple and helpful changes which can be made without too much trouble. Think, for example, about moving frequently used objects to a lower cupboard (but not too low if there is difficulty bending), choosing to use a table lamp with a more convenient switch, using a gas or electric fire rather than an open fire, and sanding down sticky drawers or doors so that they open without using excessive force. These are small changes, they cost little or nothing and they are usually easy enough to make without difficulty or causing hostility.

Special aids and equipment for kitchens and general cleaning

There are many aids available to allow easier use of the kitchen. For everyday cleaning, long-handled mops and brushes and dust-pans are invaluable and save bending. You can often buy these in large DIY stores or ironmongeries. Disposable cleaning cloths and disinfectant wipes (although expensive) save spills from rinsing cloths out. These are available in most supermarkets. A smaller washing-up bowl will weigh less when full of water than a large one. Special tap-turners can be obtained which make it easier for arthritic hands to use the taps.

Many available items make food preparation safer and easier (see Figures 1 and 2). You can get non-slip mats for placing under bowls and chopping boards, kettle tippers to obviate the need to lift a kettle full of boiling water, and grip-cloths which give a non-slip grip on the tops of jars and bottles. There are special devices available to make opening ring-pull cans easier and angled kitchen tools to do the same for food preparation. You can purchase revolving shelves to make it easier to access cupboards.

For those with limited vision, it is possible to buy packs of

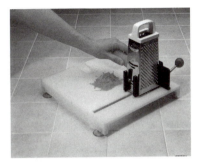

Figure 1: Cooking aid: easy-to-use chopping board and grater

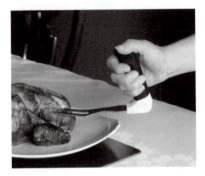

Figure 2: Angled tool: carving fork

adhesive strips or discs of brightly coloured or fluorescent material. These can be stuck around control knobs or switches, to make them easier to see. Counter tops can be edged with bright strips too.

If a major item of equipment such as a cooker or microwave oven is to be purchased it is worth giving first consideration to how easy it is to use. For example, a self-igniting gas cooker (although expensive) ensures that the gas is not left unlit by mistake. Microwave ovens are available with large figures or digits on the controls to help those with visual difficulty. Some washing machines operate by pushing a button rather than turning a dial, which may make life easier for someone with limited hand movement. Fridges especially need to be examined to see how convenient it is to reach inside and whether the

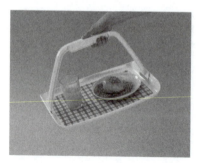

Figure 3: Tray with carrying handle

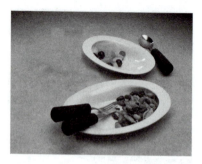

Figure 4: Adapted dishes and cutlery

shelves are contoured to make cleaning easy. There are extra-light vacuum cleaners available, or a simple carpet sweeper could be used for everyday.

There are some small items of furniture which can make a big difference to life. A step stool with a handrail can help to reach high cupboards, a perching stool will make life easier when preparing vegetables or other food, and a trolley walker which incorporates a tray eases carrying things from room to room. You can also get 'free hand' trays with a carrying handle (Figure 3), and beanbag eating trays which enable lap-top eating from a stable surface.

For eating and drinking, a whole range of specially adapted cutlery, plates and mugs are available (see Figure 4) making it easier to eat or drink one-handed or with a weak grip.

Chapter 1

Bedroom aids and equipment

The height of the bed is very important. An existing bed can be raised with special raisers but if it needs to be lower you may need to buy a new one.

****

When my Mum first equipped her cottage after Dad died it seemed clear that a high bed would make it easier for her to get in and out and at first this was ideal. What we didn't realise was that after her stroke she had real difficulty lifting her bad leg into bed and this slipped the notice of the OT assessors too. Once she told us about this we bought a lower bed as a replacement and installed a rail to help her get out of bed from the lower height.

****

You can get all sorts of backrests to make sitting up in bed more comfortable. One of the cheapest is the V-shaped pillow, which can also be used in a chair. It is very good for those who need to sleep with head and shoulders raised, and pillowcases can be bought with it for easy laundering. This pillow can be bought in many high-street stores. You can also buy rigid backrests, which will fold flat for storage, for use on a bed. Wedge shapes can be purchased to raise the foot of the bed to relieve swollen ankles. Over-bed tables can be obtained with castors which make them easy to push aside and make eating or reading in bed easier. There are also specific disability bed aids which help with sitting up or getting out of bed. The OT will advise on the best if needed.

There are various aids available to help with dressing, such as button hooks, stocking- and sock-helpers, and zip-pullers. The extent to which people find these aids helpful appears to vary widely. However, one small and simple aid for someone who finds bending difficult is the elastic shoelace. In appearance it looks like a normal lace but it enables shoes to be put on and removed without bending or difficult lace tying. You can buy these through mail order catalogues or online (see Further useful information, page 209).

Special aids and equipment in the bathroom and toilet

The bathroom is one area where there seem to be more aids and items of equipment available than in almost any other. Using these items may take time, but they do allow those with disabilities or stiffness of the limbs to be independent, and this is an area where most people wish for privacy. It is worth experimenting to find what items work best.

Bathrooms and toilets in modern houses are usually fitted with locks which can (in an emergency) be opened from the outside. These locks are also available from DIY stores and hardware shops to be fitted to existing doors and are well worth it for the carer's peace of mind.

****

My husband suffered a heart attack whilst using the toilet. Luckily I heard him fall and was able to open the bathroom lock from outside using a screwdriver. An ambulance was called by my daughter, who was visiting at the time, and he was taken to hospital and survived the attack. I was just so glad we had locks which could be opened from the outside.

****

As mentioned in the kitchen section, tap-turners are available and these can be fitted to bathroom taps for those who have trouble turning taps on and off.

There are many aids to help with washing oneself. Long-handled sponges and cloth grippers help with washing the back or the feet. Back-washing cloths with easy-to-hold handles are also available. For feet you can obtain special toe sponges which enable you to wash between your toes without bending. A towelling glove is often easier to use than a flannel for hands which cannot grip easily. Liquid soap dispensers may be easier to use than a slippery bar of soap, although you may have to test several makes to find one that is stable and does not need too much pressure to release the soap.

Walk-in showers are the ideal solution to bodily cleanliness and there are many items which can make showering easier. Grab rails will help stability when standing, and for those who find this difficult, shower stools are available which will withstand constant wetting. It is also possible to have a fixed shower-seat installed which will fold away when not in use, although this is a more expensive option. There are some designs of shower which dispense with the lip of the shower stall, but again these will have to be specially installed and may be expensive.

Many elderly people do not use a shower, either because none is installed in their accommodation or because they prefer and are used to using a bath. At the very least you should ensure that the person you are caring for has a non-slip safety mat to use in the bath. Bath rails which clip to the sides of the bath will also assist to give a safe and secure handhold. There are simple portable bath steps available which just make the task of getting in and out of the bath easier. For those who have more difficulty, there are bath boards, bath seats, and raising and lowering devices which may help. This is an area where the OT can give most helpful advice. Bath cushions will help those who find the hard surface of the bath uncomfortable.

Nearly everyone would prefer to remain independent when using the toilet. The most obvious aid in this respect is the raised toilet seat. This can be fitted in minutes and add between two and six inches to the height of the seat, which may make life considerably easier for a frail elderly person. You can also either fit grab rails next to the toilet or purchase a toilet frame which will have an adjustable height and arm rests (see Figure 5). This

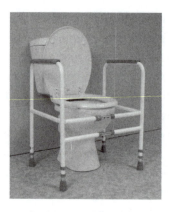

Figure 5: Raised lavatory seat with arms

makes sitting on and getting off the toilet a lot easier. Bottom-wipers are obtainable for those who have difficulty turning or reaching behind them. These are designed to hold the toilet paper and are adapted for hygienic removal of the paper after use. They will also hold moist toilet tissues and so are useful for general hygiene purposes.

It is very easy to assume that a daily bath or shower is essential and become very concerned if the person you are caring for cannot manage this. It should be remembered, however, that the daily bath or shower is a comparatively recent convention. It is possible to have a thorough all-over wash which will be as effective as a bath or shower and if this replacement for the daily bath or shower keeps your loved one happy and independent, it is worthwhile.

****

It got to the stage where Mum just couldn't manage to climb into the bath. She didn't like showers so one of us would go once a week to help her bath. On the other days she would lay a big towel over the bath mat and, standing at the basin, give herself a thorough wash using a long-handled sponge. She could manage this without help and was delighted to continue to be independent in this manner.

****

Dealing with incontinence

Issues with incontinence, specifically in dementia, are covered in Chapter 7, Dealing with dementia. However, some elderly people suffer from incontinence for physical reasons. They are aware of the problem and are able to deal with it. Doctors sometimes talk about 'urge incontinence' and 'stress incontinence'. Urge incontinence is when the sufferer has to go to the toilet in a hurry. It may happen due to weak muscular control or it may be due to diuretic medicine (sometimes known as 'water pills'). Stress incontinence happens when urine leaks out whilst the sufferer is laughing or sneezing, perhaps getting up suddenly from sitting down, or exercising. It may not matter very much which type of incontinence the person you are caring for has. You and s/he are likely to be more concerned about dealing with it on an everyday basis. All the previous suggestions about raised toilet seats and grab rails/arm rests apply here along with any other adjustments which make it quicker and easier to use the toilet. Raising the chair which is habitually used by the person, to make it quicker and easier to get up, will help, and so will making sure that s/he wears easily adjustable clothes such as loose skirts, elasticated-waist skirts and trousers, roomy pants and stockings, or pop socks rather than tights. Press-stud or Velcro fastenings, which can be undone quickly and easily, will be useful.

There is a big range of incontinence wear available, from small stick-on pads for minor leaks to fitted pads and waterproof pants. If these are needed you do not have to go to a specialist shop to get them. They are available in most supermarkets as well as from pharmacists or by mail order. If you or the person you care for are not sure what to use or buy, then consult your district nurse. In most areas there is a specialist 'Continence Advisor', who is usually a trained nurse and who can visit your cared-for and help to decide on the best way to cope with this problem. You can ask the GP or the district nurse to arrange a referral to the Continence Advisor.

General living

There are many aids available to assist independent daily living. Key-turners, which fit over the key end, will help stiff hands to turn keys. Likewise, knob- and handle-turners fit over doorhandles to make them easier to turn. Long-handled milk-bottle-holders mean that no bending is necessary to pick up the milk. Internal letter-catchers can be fitted inside the front door. Cordless phones and phones with large buttons, or large-size numbering, will make using the phone easier. Mobile phones are now available with large, easy-to-use keys and simple instructions. Special loops can be fitted to electric plugs to make them easier to grip, or you can obtain cheaper add-on or stick-on devices. An electrician can raise the most used sockets so that no bending is required to reach them. Special smoke alarms and door- and telephone-bells can be purchased which flash instead of sounding for the hard of hearing. It goes without saying that remote controls for TV, DVD and music centres will make life easier and all of these can be bought with larger-than-normal buttons to make them easier to see and use.

Raising the person you are caring for's favourite chair may make a big difference to her/him when it comes to standing up and sitting down, and it is possible to buy inexpensive chair-raisers for this purpose. If affordable, a rising/reclining chair will make life even easier. These can be manually or electrically operated and will help someone who has stiffness or who is unsteady to stand up in a controlled manner. They are very expensive to buy new as they are often made to order. However, you can try to obtain one second hand.

Safety

When it comes to safety, a simple door chain costs very little, is easy to fit and will give reassurance when answering the front door. (However, if carers or visitors normally let themselves in with a key, then your cared-for must not leave the chain in place all the time. You could put a sign up by the door to remind her / him to use the door chain before answering the door themselves.) A TV security camera can be bought for quite a small expense and fitted via the TV to allow someone living alone to view who is at the door before they even open it.

Outside lights with sensors which come on if someone ap-proaches the house are simple to fit and not very expensive.

Personal alarms are very useful if the person you care for is liable to fall or to need help when out of reach of a telephone. These usually have a central unit, and help can be obtained by pressing a button on this unit. They also incorporate a satellite unit which the user can wear as a bracelet or a pendant. A permanently-staffed call centre will answer if the button is pressed and will either advise the person what to do next or will call out the best helper – the carer or the emergency services, for example. Unfortunately these alarms are not a good solution if the user is so safety conscious regarding electric sockets that s/he might inadvertently switch off or unplug the unit, or if s/he suffers from dementia and cannot understand or learn what to do in an emergency. Also, there are many elderly people who object to wearing the alarm, though some modern ones are relatively small and can more easily be hidden under the user's clothes. You will need to discuss with the person you are caring for whether this is the most appropriate emergency aid for her/him.

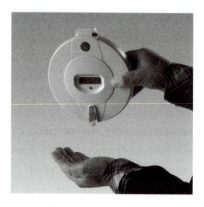

Figure 6: Pivotell's advance pill dispenser

Medicines are usually dispensed in bottles with child-resistant caps, but you can ask at the pharmacy for an ordinary screw-top bottle. 'Organisers' for pills, which help the elderly person to remember to take their medicines on time, are available – some very simple, some very sophisticated (Figure 6). The pharmacist will be able to advise about these and to supply medication in ready-made-up 'blister packs' to make life easier. For those who have trouble swallowing pills, it may be possible to have a liquid alternative. It is important to ask the doctor about this if it is needed, because the doctor may not even think of this eventuality.

Huge strides have been made in electronic remote-care options for elderly or frail people. Known as 'telecare' and 'telehealth' technology, there are now a number of systems available to assist with monitoring health and safety. Some can monitor such things as blood pressure and blood glucose levels; some are pressure-pad systems which alert a carer if, for example, the person s/he is caring for does not return to bed after visiting the toilet (perhaps because s/he has had a fall), or monitor when the front door is opened. Not all systems are useful for those who have dementia, but these options are well worth looking into.

In the garden

If the person you are caring for is a keen gardener, there are a multitude of aids available to help her/him enjoy their garden. Strangely enough, many of the best aids will be found in specialist gardening catalogues rather than in 'disabled' equipment catalogues.

Many simple adaptations to the garden will help, such as raised flower beds, extended patio/hardstanding areas and pot raisers.

For those who suffer from a specific disability, any of the appropriate organisations which offer support in that area will be able to offer more specific information about aids and equipment. For example, many aids are specifically designed for those who are blind, partially sighted or deaf, and these may not be available through general disability centres or shops and catalogues.

Finding and obtaining aids and equipment

This chapter has been written to give general advice about the help, in the form of aids and equipment, which is available. It is unfortunately not possible to give specific advice in a general work of this nature. Items of equipment can be obtained from many suppliers. Some things are free via the health service or social services and some are available for hire at low cost through organisations like the Red Cross or through charities. You may like to do initial research via the internet and then follow this up by seeing the equipment and trying it out. There are Disabled Living Centres and shops in many towns, where items can be examined and tried out and where assistance and advice is on hand to help you decide what to purchase. A great many things can be purchased through local pharmacies. Some sources of supply are listed in this chapter's Further useful information section (see end of book). If money is short, it is also worth investigating what is available locally, either free or on long-term loan. Many local councils offer lending schemes, and churches and other local charity groups may offer renovated second-hand equipment.

Chapter 2

Financial matters – including benefits and entitlements

My mother could cope perfectly well with all her everyday living needs but she had never managed the finances – apart from the cash sum my father passed to her for housekeeping purposes. She was sound in her mind and able to understand money matters but had never dealt with banks, chequebooks or cashcards (and did not want to learn how to). She wanted me and my brother to do that part for her.

****

This chapter looks at ways in which you as a carer might help the relative or friend you are caring for with managing her/his finances. A significant section covers Lasting Power of Attorney. Making arrangements to cover fees for care or nursing homes is discussed and there is also some information about various benefits and entitlements.

There are still many partnerships where only one of the partners takes charge of the everyday management of money and following the death of the spouse who did that, the other may view the prospect of taking on the handling of bank statements, chequebooks, standing orders, direct debits and debit/credit cards with dismay. How you help to resolve this will depend upon your relationship with that person, of course. Some people will need just a little help with understanding how financial institutions work and others will want to hand the entire 'package' over to someone else.

If the person you care for develops dementia, then it is likely that at some stage s/he will become unable to manage her/his finances and will need help, perhaps on a daily basis.

Dealing with joint bank accounts following a bereavement

If the person you care for had a joint account with her/his partner then, as discussed in Chapter 13, it is easily converted on the death of one partner into the sole name of the survivor. If s/he has not been used to handling a bank account and wants help, then it might be worth discussing at this stage the possibility of transferring the account into joint names with you, her/his carer. You can arrange for all actions on the account (including paying by cheque) to need both account signatures or you can arrange that the signature of either one of you is sufficient. Dual signatures might reassure someone who wants to feel in control of their money but single either/or signatures may make it simpler if the person you care for is ever unavailable (for example, in hospital) to sign when necessary. If you do not bank with the same bank as the person you care for, then the bank will want to see proof of your identity when you convert the account, just as if you were opening an account in your sole name.

Savings accounts and securities

Usually, savings accounts and securities can also be put into joint names and again the best time to do this is when the account name has to be changed anyway. The procedures will be similar to changing to a joint bank account and any financial institution will want various proofs of identity from you as above.

Benefits payments

If the person you are caring for is in receipt of benefits that are normally paid into her/his bank or building society account and s/he is unable to collect cash from that account on a temporary basis, s/he can write to the bank or building society, asking them to give temporary power to someone else to operate her/his account (see above). If any payments are normally paid by cheque, s/he can fill in the back of the cheque to allow someone else to cash it for them. The benefits office is usually very helpful if the person you care for wants you to be able to act for them and discuss problems about benefits.

Power of Attorney

Power of Attorney (POA) is a legal process in which someone (the 'donor') hands over to someone else (the 'attorney') power to decide what is done with their finances and property. An 'Enduring Power of Attorney' (EPA) could previously be used to authorise an attorney (generally a relative or friend) to carry out all tasks for the donor. Enduring Power of Attorney can no longer be granted; it has been superseded by 'Lasting Power of Attorney'. However, if the person you are caring for has an EPA in place which was drawn up before November 2007, it is still perfectly legal. You DO NOT have to replace it with a Lasting Power of Attorney unless you wish to make 'welfare' (non-financial) decisions for your cared-for. Many people have been put to unnecessary extra expense by listening to wrong advice in this respect.

It is always a good idea to consider making a POA so that someone you trust can manage your financial (and if desired, your welfare) affairs if the necessity arises. Many people put off doing this 'until it is necessary'. However, none of us can see the future. A POA can only be given if you have the mental capacity to understand the full implications. It needs to be signed and witnessed. If you are unable (due to being incapacitated) to 'give' the POA, no one can do so on your behalf without recourse to a complicated application to the Court of Protection (see below). If you develop dementia and are unable to understand what giving a POA means, then you will not be able to appoint a person of your choosing to look after your finances.

Anyone can make a Lasting Power of Attorney (LPA), but in order to do so, as I have said, a person needs to be mentally capable of making the decision to take this step and if you are using a solicitor s/he will not go ahead unless s/he is sure of this. If the person you are caring for is not mentally capable of making a LPA, again, see the section below on the Court of Protection.

The person you are caring for can give her/his 'attorney' (the person to whom s/he is entrusting her/his finances) complete power over her/his financial affairs or s/he can put restrictions on that power. For example, s/he can specify that her/his attorney cannot sell her/his house without permission.

The forms to set up a LPA can be obtained from the Court of Protection or downloaded from their website: www.gov.uk/power-of-attorney. There is also a very helpful booklet available from the Court of Protection, which explains the LPA and the procedure for setting it up. The Court of Protection makes it clear that you do not have to use a solicitor to set up the LPA.

You are likely to find, however, that the people you deal with in banks and financial institutions are unaware of this rule. They are likely to demand that the document is signed and sealed by a solicitor. You may therefore decide that it is easier to use a solicitor to make the arrangements in the first place, although this will increase the cost.

Enduring Power of Attorney

The following section applies if an EPA was set up before November 2007. The rules are different for LPAs, so skip to the next section as relevant.

Chapter 2

****

My mother set up an EPA naming me as the attorney. We lodged the document with the solicitor who had helped set it up for safe-keeping, but years later when we wanted a certified copy to give to the bank he refused to send me one. We wrote and telephoned several times but he said that he was not able to release the document without my mother's agreement. As my mother was suffering from dementia by then, we wanted to lodge the EPA with the Court of Protection and even they could not understand why the solicitor wouldn't give us the document. Eventually, he only handed over the EPA when the Court of Protection threatened to intervene directly. If we had to do this again I would retain the document myself.

****

Whether you use a solicitor or not, it may be advisable for either you or the person you are caring for to retain the signed document yourself in a safe place. Banks will not keep the original copy for their records but they will not accept a photocopy made by you. You will need to take the document into the bank and let them make a copy which they will certify as a true copy and retain for their records. If the person you care for loses her/his mental capacity and you hold an EPA, then you must register it with the Public Guardianship Office (PGO) (or Office of Care and Protection in Northern Ireland). You have an absolute duty to do so, and you may not use the Enduring Power of Attorney until you have applied to register it. After you have applied to register the EPA, but before the registration actually happens (it can take a while because the PGO has to wait to see if anyone objects) you will have limited authority to maintain the donor and prevent loss to her/his estate.

Before you apply to register the EPA, you should give notice of your intention to do so to the donor and to the donor's nearest relatives. This is because the donor and her/his relatives are entitled to object to the registration of the power or to you as the attorney. There are standard forms that you must use and certain classes of people whom you have to notify. For example, if you notify one child of the donor you must notify all children. The PGO will supply the forms you need (or you can download them from the relevant website (www.gov.uk/power-of-attorney) together with exact instructions about notifying and registering.

You also have to certify that you have notified the donor, even if s/he is unable to understand the notification. You send the notification forms to those who should be notified and there is then a period of time in which they can object to the appointment of the nominated attorney. However, the PGO is not likely to accept a frivolous objection and would want substantial reasons why you should not be appointed since you were the person your cared-for wished to appoint as attorney when signing the EPA.

There is, of course, a fee to be paid for registration of the EPA, but this can be paid from your cared-for's funds.

If there are no objections (or if the PGO overrules the objections), the EPA is returned to you signed and sealed. This signed EPA must now be registered with all the financial institutions where the person you are caring for has accounts. You do not need to (and should not) part with the registered EPA. Take it physically to each institution and they will make a 'certified photocopy'. If the person you are caring for holds postal building society or electronic accounts, then contact the institution to find out the procedure. Normally you can have a certified copy made at a local high-street branch of the relevant institution for forwarding on.

Lasting Power of Attorney

The rules for a Lasting Power of Attorney are different. A LPA has to be registered with the Court of Protection before it can be used.

If the person you are caring for becomes mentally incapacitated and no LPA is in place you have to notify the Court of Protection of this fact. The Court of Protection will then appoint someone to manage her/his affairs. Often this is a relative or family member, but the court may appoint someone else. It is very important therefore to consider with the person you care for the matter of giving power of attorney in good time and whilst s/he still has mental capacity.

POA in practice

Banks and building societies differ in their procedures. Some will just note the EPA /LPA in their records and some will close the accounts in your cared-for's name and open new ones entitled, for example, 'J Smith POA for Mrs M Smith'. If this is the case, new cheque- or passbooks will be issued for the account. Many banks will not allow a cash (debit) card on POA accounts, which may make it more difficult for you to manage the affairs of your cared-for. It is difficult to understand the reasons for this since you can of course draw cash by signing a cheque on the account whenever required.

****

When we registered the POA for my mother-in-law, the bank withdrew her debit card and would not issue one on the new account. When I enquired why, I was told that it was because, due to her mental incapacity, she might 'draw out all her money'. When I pointed out that it was her money and she was entitled to do so they didn't really have any answer. They promised to write to me with an explanation but never did so.

****

Once you have registered the POA it is best to keep careful records of your management of your cared-for's money. The Court can ask to see your records at any time, although they seldom do so. You also have a duty to keep your cared-for's money and financial affairs separate from your own. You now have the power to set up and cancel direct debits and standing orders on behalf of the person you are caring for (see Chapter 13 for information about paying utilities by direct debit), to write cheques and to withdraw cash and spend it for her/his benefit. You also have the power to make cash gifts if this is something s/he would normally do. For example, if Granny always gave a Christmas present of cash to her grandchildren you can make similar gifts on her behalf from her funds. However, you should be careful to use your cared-for's money in a responsible manner in accordance with the instructions given by the PGO when granting the registration.

An EPA may appear to give wide-ranging powers, but you should note that they are purely financial. For example, you may be able to claim benefits on behalf of the person you are caring for, but you cannot make medical decisions for her/him. You do not have the right to decide where s/he should live (although in practice, because you manage her/his financial affairs, you may be able to do so). You cannot make a Will on her/his behalf, nor change a Will which s/he had made at an earlier date. Perhaps surprisingly, you cannot nominate another attorney if you no longer feel able to carry out these duties. If you wish to relinquish your POA, the Court will nominate another attorney. (In practice they usually nominate a close relative but it may not be the one of your choosing.) The point is that it was the person you are caring for who chose the attorney and you cannot change her/his decision.

A Lasting Power of Attorney on the other hand comes in two parts: one part for property and financial affairs and the other part for health and welfare affairs. The person you are caring for can give Power of Attorney for just one part or for both parts. If you hold a LPA for the health and welfare affairs of the person you are caring for, then you can make decisions in these areas. Full guidance is available from the Office of the Public Guardian.

Paying nursing home fees

I knew that my mother would probably have to fund part of her nursing home fees but frankly I was horrified to realise how expensive these would be and, of course, we had no idea how long the funding would be needed for. We consulted a specialist financial advisor. One of the surprising things was that Mum could invest a lump sum and be assured of her fees being covered for as long as she lived. She found it hard to make the decision to use such a large sum, but in the event she (and we) did achieve peace of mind for the last seven years of her life. We were happier to see her use the money to ensure her own comfort than to try to save it to pass on to us.

****

When and if the time comes to consider moving to a residential care home or a nursing home, the person you are caring for, like many older people today, may not meet the criteria for state financial assistance for care/nursing home fees. Alternatively, they may choose to enter a care home independently of any state aid. However, her/his available capital, perhaps savings or the proceeds from the sale of a former home, if left in a high-interest deposit account, may not yield sufficient income to meet the high costs involved. Consequently, many people find their money runs out long before their need for care ceases. But there are specialist care-fees advisors who can help with planning for care home costs. You and the person you are caring for may find it useful to consult one of these.

How can a care-fees advisor help? Firstly, a competent advisor who understands the complexities of Local and Health Authority support, DWP benefits, tax efficiency and legal arrangements can ensure you and the person you are caring for are aware of your proper entitlements. Secondly, such advisory firms will provide the person you are caring for with appropriate financial advice so that s/he can afford her/his chosen type of care.

The financial products that are appropriate for meeting care costs vary according to an individual's age, health, required income and the degree of risk a family is prepared to take. Proper advisors aim to identify financial products that deliver returns significantly above those provided by deposit-based savings, but without taking undue risks with capital. It is worth consulting such an advisor if it is clear that the person you are caring for may need nursing home care in the future.

Ideal financial products are those that can provide a regular income and incorporate flexibility to meet any future changes in care needs – for example, fee increases or the additional cost of moving from a residential care home to a nursing home. The ultimate aim might be to enable care costs to be met for the life of the person you are caring for whilst, as far as possible, preserving original capital, independence and, if s/he wishes, as many people do, the ability to leave an inheritance.

Good questions to ask a financial advisor about a financial product concerned with care/nursing home fees are:

1. Does the product provide fees indefinitely or only for a limited number of years?
2. Does the product provide for increases in fees?
3. How much will my cared-for need to invest?
4. Will this product give more security than a simple investment of the funds available?

Benefits and entitlements

The district nurse advised me to find out if my mother could claim the Attendance Allowance. Whist I was researching that I discovered that I could claim Carer's Allowance myself as I had left my job in order to look after Mum. This led me to search

Chapter 2

further and I found a whole range of entitlements which Mum could get and which we hadn't even known about.

****

Many people fail to take full advantage of state support or make decisions to claim or not to claim without fully appreciating the consequences. There are a number of different benefits to which the person you are caring for might be entitled. Some are listed below with a short description of the circumstances in which they can be claimed. The whole benefits area is very complicated and sometimes you can actually end up worse off overall because you claim a certain benefit. The list that follows is only meant to give you a starting point to investigate what might be available. Telephone helpline and website addresses are given at the end of the book where possible to help you with further research. The Citizens Advice Bureau can also help. In fact, 'benefits advice' is one of the major reasons the public give for consulting the CAB.

In order to apply for most benefits you will have to complete application forms, but most have been designed to be as simple and easy to understand as possible. In some cases you can complete and sign the forms on behalf of the person you are caring for. Most forms can be completed online.

Welfare reform changes start in 2013. Many existing means-tested benefits will eventually be abolished and replaced by a new benefits system. Therefore it is important that anyone concerned about benefits and allowances available for someone they care for should consult an up-to-date guide. The CAB has an 'advice guide' to benefits on their website (www.citizensadvice.org.uk) which is easy to search and which contains information pertaining to England, Scotland, Wales and Northern Ireland.

Age-related benefits

Age-related benefits include the following:
- Pension credit
- Housing credit
- Council tax benefit (this is one of the benefits changing from 2013)
- Over-80 pension – a state pension for people aged 80 or over who have little or no state pension. Unlike other state pensions, it is not based on National Insurance contributions.

Disability and caring-related benefits

- **Carer's Allowance** – A taxable benefit for informal carers aged 16 or over spending at least 35 hours a week looking after someone who is getting or waiting to hear about Attendance Allowance, Disability Living Allowance, or Constant Attendance Allowance.
- **Disability Living Allowance** – This is being replaced by the new Personal Independence Payment from 2013, on a phased basis. Eventually, it will replace Disability Living Allowance (DLA) for all new claims and for existing DLA claimants who are aged 16 to 64 on 8 April 2013, or who reach age 16 after 8 April 2013.
- **Attendance Allowance** – This is paid if you need help to look after yourself, and/or if you become ill or disabled on or after your 65th birthday, or are claiming on or after your 65th birthday. It is paid at different rates depending on whether you need care during the day, during the night, or both.

Chapter 2

Heating and energy use

The following two schemes should not be confused:

- **Winter Fuel Payments** – You will automatically get Winter Fuel Payment if you are aged 60 or over and live in the UK and are in receipt of the State Pension.
- **Cold Weather Payments** – These help people on a low income with fuel costs during periods of cold weather. Cold weather payments are different from Winter Fuel Payments which are made every winter to people over state pension age, regardless of the temperature.

Housing and general living benefits for those on a low income

- **Housing benefit** (under the new rules there is a 'cap' on this benefit and it will eventually be replaced by Universal credit)
- **Council tax benefit/reduction**
- **Council tax disregard** – This is available if the person you are caring for suffers from dementia or other 'severe mental impairment'. It is not the same as council tax benefit/reduction; essentially, the council will 'disregard' the person concerned when assessing for council tax payment.

Social and entertainment

- **Free TV Licence** – If the person you are caring for is aged 75 or over, s/he is entitled to a free television licence. If s/he is 74, you can apply for a short-term licence to cover the months until s/he reaches 75. S/he can also get TV licence concessions if s/he is living in residential care.

Chapter 3

Getting about

This chapter looks at the problems with, and solutions to, getting about for generally-able elderly persons. The discussion covers the frail, less mobile and easily tired elderly. If the person you care for has a specific long-term disability, specialist advice is needed; there may be an association or specialist health therapist who can advise you about her/his needs. For this reason, wheelchairs and electric scooters are not covered at length here.

Getting about is often a problem even for the fit elderly and you as a carer may be heavily involved in this aspect of your cared-for's daily life. The problems incurred, and their solutions, fall into different categories depending upon whether your relative/friend is a car driver or uses public transport. This chapter also considers problems related to walking and general mobility. As I repeat throughout this book, do not rely solely on information and aid from 'official' sources. Many local groups and charities offer support and help in individual cases. Your local library and the internet are the best sources of information about this. It may be particularly worth contacting any charity or voluntary organisation linked to the profession to which the person you care for may belong or have belonged. Several of these organisations are listed in the reference section at the end of the book.

Driving

Driving licences have to be renewed at three-yearly intervals for those over the age of 70 years. Those who hold a driving licence will automatically be sent a reminder application form by the DVLA 90 days before their 70th birthday. This form must be completed ensuring that all the relevant questions are answered. The person you care for will need to enclose original documentation confirming her/his identity, and a passport-style colour photograph if her/his licence is an old-style 'paper' licence. Holders of a photocard licence will not need to provide documentation or a photo. You can also renew your licence online at www.gov.uk/renew-your-driving-licence-if-you-are-70-or-over.

The likely reality is that the elderly relative/friend you are caring for will be over the age of 70 and will already be in the three-year renewal cycle. Sometimes the DVLA requires a report or an examination by a GP, or even a specialist doctor. Doctors are entitled to make a charge for a medical report or a medical examination and they are required to list their charges for these services in a public area of the General Practice premises. Most GPs are sympathetic to the needs of their elderly patients and many will not charge them even though they are entitled to do so. If the person you care for would find difficulty in paying it is always worth approaching the GP practice to request that they waive the charge.

It is worth checking that the person you are caring for is not paying out needlessly for certain other items. For example, s/he is exempt from paying the Vehicle Excise Duty (Road Tax) if s/he receives:

- The higher rate of the mobility component of the Disability Living Allowance

or

- War Pensioners' Mobility Supplement.

If s/he is eligible for these exemptions but is not able to drive her/himself, s/he may nominate another person's vehicle (for example yours) to be exempted from tax. To qualify for exemption the vehicle should be used substantially for the purposes of the disabled person.

If the person you are caring for gets the higher rate of the mobility component of the Disability Living Allowance, or War Pensioners' Mobility Supplement, s/he should automatically be sent the exemption forms. Otherwise you or s/he can contact the DVLA for details, or see their website (www.dvla.gov.uk).

The Blue Badge scheme

The main purpose of the Blue Badge scheme is to allow disabled and blind people to park, or be parked, closer to their destination. The scheme does not necessarily allow a vehicle to park free of charge. When a vehicle is parked, the Blue Badge should be displayed so that the holder's name and the date of expiry are visible. The person entitled to have a badge may be a driver or a passenger. This means that you could display the badge on your car if you are driving the person you care for.

The Blue Badge generally means that you can:

- Park without charge or time limit at parking meters
- Park without time limit in streets where waiting is allowed for limited periods
- Park on single- or double-yellow lines for up to three hours. In Scotland there is no time limit
- Park in designated 'Blue Badge' disabled parking spaces in public car parks.

However, a Blue Badge is not a licence to park just anywhere. Some restrictions do apply and the above is for guidance only. For example, you cannot park in bus lanes, cycle lanes, when loading restrictions apply, etc. You will need to read the full instructions that you or your cared-for receives with the Blue Badge.

It is an offence to display a Blue Badge if the disabled person has not been in the vehicle prior to its being parked, unless the driver is parking to collect the disabled person. So you should not have the badge on display whilst you are using the car solely for your own requirements.

The person you care for can obtain a Blue Badge without further assessment if he or she:

- is registered blind
- receives War Pensioners' Mobility Supplement
- receives the higher rate of the mobility component of the Disability Living Allowance (DLA)
- receives the mobility component of the Personal Independence Payment (PIP) and scored at least 8 points in relation to the 'moving around' activity in the PIP assessment
- has been awarded a lump sum benefit from the Armed Forces Compensation scheme (tariffs 1 to 8). Has also been certified as having a permanent or substantial disability which means s/he can't walk or finds walking very difficult
- receives a government grant towards her/his own vehicle.

Contact your local council or apply via www.gov.uk/apply-blue-badge. Local councils' rules may vary slightly. Be aware, the GP may be asked for medical evidence about the degree of disability.

If the person you are caring for does not hold a Blue Badge you may still feel that s/he (or you if you are driving her/him) should be able to park in a disabled bay because, for example, s/he has difficulty in walking the distance from the normal car parking spaces to the relevant shop or amenity. You or s/he should not park in a designated Blue Badge space unless the car has a Blue Badge displayed. However, some shops and car parks have spaces which are labelled 'for disabled use' and not specifically for Blue Badge holders. Most shops and supermarkets will be sympathetic if you use these spaces to save the person you care for a tiring walk.

Holding a driving licence does not necessarily mean that you are fit to drive. Vision problems may get worse over the years but may not have been noticed and so may not have been reported to, or recorded by, the GP. Minor strokes may have occurred and not been recognised. Movement in the limbs may have been affected to a degree which makes it unsafe to drive. This is one of the most difficult areas for carers. On the one hand, the ownership of a car and the ability to drive confer a huge element of independence on the person you are caring for. You as a carer are also relieved of the problem of arranging transport for everyday activities. On the other hand, driving (even locally and over well known routes) is an activity fraught with danger if undertaken by someone who is not medically fit to drive, and the danger is not just to the driver but to other road users and pedestrians.

****

My mother only used the car to do her local shopping and go to the hairdresser and so on. She was always driving on familiar territory and I didn't think there was a problem. But one day she had a minor bump in a car park and hit her head. She then abandoned the car and was found by the police wandering around the shopping centre. When we talked it over it became clear that she shouldn't be driving any longer. The police said that they would not prosecute provided we sent her licence back to the DVLA and that she didn't drive again. She was 81 at the time.

****

If you are not sure whether someone you care for is fit to drive, look out for the following signs:
- Driving at inappropriate speeds, either too fast or too slowly
- Asking passengers to help check if it is clear to turn left or right
- Responding slowly to or not noticing pedestrians, cyclists and other drivers

- Ignoring, disobeying or misinterpreting street signs and traffic lights
- Failing to judge distances between cars correctly – for example, driving too close to the vehicle in front
- Having one or more near accidents or near misses
- Drifting across lane markings or bumping into curbs
- Forgetting to turn on headlights when they are needed
- Having difficulty with glare from oncoming headlights and streetlights, especially at dawn and dusk
- Finding it difficult to turn to look over her/his shoulder to reverse
- Losing the way in normally familiar routes.

If someone has a diagnosis of dementia they have a legal duty to inform the DVLA of this fact. Failure to inform the DVLA may invalidate any motor insurance and may incur a fine. The DVLA does not necessarily revoke the driving licence immediately – many people with dementia are still fit to drive – but it may ask for further information from the GP of the person concerned.

It may be very difficult to persuade the person you care for that s/he should stop driving, but if s/he becomes unfit to drive or decides to give up it is not all bad news. For one thing, sale of the vehicle may bring in a useful capital sum. There is no longer a need to worry about servicing and repairs and insurance policies, and roadside rescue agreements can be cancelled. If you are a driver yourself, the person you care for may opt to keep the car and have the insurance changed to your name so that you can have use of the vehicle to take her/him out when required.

Alternatives to driving

When my mother-in-law could no longer use the car she agreed to let my son have it on permanent loan on condition that he drove her out on errands or to the local shops etc. We had to ensure that he understood that a condition of the loan was that he gave his grandmother's needs priority, but overall we all benefited from the arrangement. There were fewer calls on our time, he gained the use of a car which he would not otherwise have been able to afford and in fact he became, over time, very fond of his little excursions with her.

****

At this stage you might give consideration to what needs the person you care for has which actually require some form of transport. Often you can cut the need for transport to a minimum with a few lifestyle changes. For example, most doctors' surgeries will send completed prescription forms to the pharmacist of your choice and many pharmacists will deliver the made-up prescription free to your friend/relative's house. Most large supermarkets offer an online ordering service and home-delivery of groceries and household articles. If your relative/friend cannot use a computer you can make the order on her/his behalf. This is very convenient as heavy shopping is delivered right to the door at a time of your/her/his choice. Mail order shopping continues to be an expanding area, either through catalogues which come to the door or via web pages – virtually anything can now be ordered without leaving home.

Of course, the person you care for will not want to be confined to the house unnecessarily, and getting about without a car is now much easier for elderly people thanks to the many local council schemes in operation. Contact your local council to see what they offer. In particular, ask about the following:

Local bus travel

Local travel for elderly people is now free in many areas (usually outside the rush hour), but you will have to find out how this operates in your locality. Some local authorities offer tokens which can be used on buses and in parking meters and are often accepted by local taxi firms. Others issue a renewable pass which needs to be produced for each journey. If the person you are caring for is still mobile and lives in an urban area, then local buses may be of immense use. Routes nearly always operate from outlying areas into town centres to allow for shopping. Frequently the buses will stop 'on request' to allow passengers to alight near home, and local drivers may come to know their regular passengers well and be prepared to help with parcels and shopping. Many public vehicles also now have wheelchair and 'lift' access for those who find climbing steps difficult. In rural areas the bus services may be less frequent but many small outlying communities now benefit from local enterprise in the form of 'post buses' or special transport laid on with the elderly non-driver in mind. In many areas, both in town and country, special buses are arranged and paid for by large superstores to allow shoppers to come to them. Most large hospitals also have some sort of shuttle bus service from outlying areas. Where local post offices have recently been closed down, local councils have sometimes arranged for special buses to be run to enable customers to reach the nearest post office from small villages or outlying areas. Find out about these and similar arrangements by contacting your local authority or your local library.

Telephone booking buses (Dial-a-ride)
This type of arrangement (there are a variety of descriptive titles depending on where you live) is sometimes operated by the local council, either through a contracted service or sometimes by volunteers. These services provide door-to-door transport for anyone who finds it difficult or impossible to use ordinary public transport. You don't have to be registered disabled or confined to a wheelchair to use such services – for example, you might have difficulty climbing steps on buses, or be unable to walk to the bus

stop. Dial-a-ride-type service vehicles can also carry passengers in wheelchairs. Fares are about the same as you would pay on ordinary buses. You will need to book journeys well in advance to be sure of a seat. The person concerned will be collected from her/his door at the arranged time, and the driver will help her/him into the vehicle. Usually vehicles are equipped with a lift or ramp, which can be used by anyone who has difficulty in climbing steps.

A number of voluntary organisations, both locally and nationally, provide transport for individuals in various areas. In most cases, these services rely on volunteer drivers who may be reimbursed a mileage rate when using their own car. Passengers will generally be asked to contribute towards the cost of this transport, although rates will vary between organisations. The type of service provided is often confined to lifts to doctors' surgeries or to local hospitals for outpatient clinics. Details of these volunteer services can usually be obtained via your local council or from your local library. Volunteers will sometimes also provide an escort service into the outpatients department if, for example, the person you are caring for is unable to cope alone.

Train travel

Most train companies have arrangements for disabled passengers and this may include those who just need a little extra help to get on and off trains or find the right connections. The train companies can usually arrange for staff to meet your cared-for at her/his departure station, accompany her/him to the train and see her/him safely on board. Similar arrangements can be made at the destination station and other stations if there is a need to change trains. For example, ramps can be provided for wheelchair users or wheelchairs between platforms for those who are mobile but cannot walk far. You will need to contact the individual train companies to find out details. Sometimes you can obtain details at the local station ticket office but often you may find you have to ring a special 'enquiries' number. Most train companies are better able to help if you contact them as far in advance of the journey as possible. Look on individual websites or contact train companies by phone or enquire at local stations' ticket offices.

Taxis

If your local council provides tokens instead of bus passes, these are often accepted in payment by taxi services. Many taxi services are extending their fleet of vehicles now to include cars with ramps or let-down steps to make it easier for elderly and disabled persons to use them. The local council usually carries details of taxi firms with facilities for the disabled on its website or you can get this information in leaflet form at the local library. Businesses such as hairdressers and restaurants will usually agree to telephone for a taxi for their customers to return home after an appointment and may know which taxi services are most helpful to the elderly or disabled.

Local informal arrangements

Don't feel that you have to find 'official' transport for your cared-for. Often friends and neighbours are happy to help out with a lift to the shops, to a lunch club or to a day centre. If the person you care for is a regular churchgoer, a word with the vicar, priest or minister will usually ensure that a lift to church can be arranged with another parishioner as nearly all churches operate some sort of lift/shared transport scheme. Similarly, if your cared-for regularly attends a local club or association and is no longer able to drive to meetings, an approach to the organisation will often result in the offer of a lift to meetings.

Visiting shops and other amenities

Elderly people, although not actually disabled, may tire easily or simply be very frail. They may enjoy outings and visits but need extra help in getting about or finding articles on sale, or simply need to sit down frequently. Most large supermarkets and garden centres now supply free loans of wheelchairs for customers who need them. If the wheelchairs are not obviously on view it is always worth asking if they are available. Some shops may not be able to keep them near the entrance. (There is even a growing trade in stealing wheelchairs from store entrances so some traders may prefer to keep them under supervision when not in use.)

Tourist attractions, such as stately homes, gardens and cathedrals, also have wheelchairs for hire or free loan. If you are planning a visit it may be worth telephoning in advance to reserve a wheelchair where this is allowed. Smaller shops and businesses now have, by law, to make suitable concessions to help those who are disabled or less mobile. This may mean that they simply display a notice saying that they will give assistance if asked. Take advantage of the law and do so! Most shops will supply a chair for frail customers to sit down, for example. Larger supermarkets often provide an accompanied shopping service where a member of staff will walk around the store with a less able person and reach things from high/low shelves and carry the shopping basket. The biggest obstacle you may encounter when trying to arrange such help is resistance from the person you care for. S/he may hate to be seen as 'disabled' or in need of help.

****

My mother suffered from heart failure and got out of breath very easily. She could walk, but not far and only very slowly. It was frustrating for her and for us because she loved shopping and visiting local attractions but kept denying any need to use a wheelchair. One day she visited my sister for a few days and my sister informed her that she had hired a wheelchair for her to use 'just so that you can visit the cathedral'. Mum loved old churches and accepted this suggestion as a 'one-off'. After this she was converted and happily chose to use free wheelchairs when visiting big stores and the local garden centre.

****

Personal comfort

Elderly people may need to use the toilet more often than others. Not all public toilets are open when needed and most do not have facilities (raised toilet seats, for example) that the person you care for may need. A very useful scheme is operated by RADAR (Royal Association for Disability and Rehabilitation – now Disability Rights UK) whereby you can write to them with your cared-for's details and they will supply, for a nominal cost, a key which opens the locks of around 4000 disabled toilets in car parks and public places throughout the UK. You have to put the request in writing in order to explain why your cared-for needs the key but s/he does not have to be registered disabled to apply – having stiffness from arthritis, for example, is sufficient. This is an extremely useful amenity. Many elderly and disabled people avoid leaving home even if they would enjoy an outing because they are afraid they will need the toilet at inappropriate times.

Walking aids

There are now many types of walking aid available. If you need a walking aid you are entitled to a free assessment. This is available by arrangement through your GP, and sometimes supplies of equipment are free, so before buying any kind of walking aid, be it stick, frame or rollator trolley, it is important to arrange for a professional assessment. The assessment will confirm the most suitable walking aid needed, the correct height or type, and any particular adaptations required.

Walking sticks

The varnished wooden stick is attractive and traditional. However, many different designs of walking stick are now available. For example, you can get a stick with a 'crutch-type' armrest for someone who needs this. Also available is a 'Fischer' stick with a handle for a more comfortable grip for people who have arthritis or difficulty with their hands. You can also get sticks with a tripod foot for greater stability. A tight grip is required to gain support from a walking stick, so these are only suitable for people who are still reasonably mobile and strong. Sticks should also be of the correct height and should have the ferrule / rubber tip checked for wear at regular intervals. If you are unsure, your local physiotherapy department will give advice on the best type of walking stick for each individual; you may have to get a referral to the physiotherapist through the GP or district nurse.

Walking frames

There are two main varieties of walking frame – a 'box-style' frame with rigid legs, and a frame with two front wheels to allow easier movement. The classic box-style 'Zimmer' is very stable and easily gripped, but it requires two hands and is cumbersome to transport. These products have been so dominant as aids for the elderly that the 'Zimmer', just like the 'Hoover', has become a household name. There are, however, many different types of walking aid available now which make the traditional 'Zimmer' seem almost archaic.

Trolleys

You can obtain shopping trolleys which have an added seat and this is ideal for someone who gets tired easily but is otherwise able to get about and do her / his own shopping. S / he can place purchases inside the carrier, and rest on the padded top for a short time if walking becomes too tiring.

Rollators

Rollators have wheels which allow you to turn and pivot in a way that trolleys cannot. Rollators are a lightweight yet sturdy walker alternative. There are many different types. Four-wheeled models (see Figure 7) are a better option for use on uneven ground and outdoors, but three-wheeled models are more manoeuvrable indoors. It may be best to look through a catalogue or check the various websites before deciding on the one for your cared-for. An even better solution is to visit a showroom and try out various models. However, if this is not possible, almost all vendors operate a postal order and delivery service, often with next-day delivery. In general they are very reasonably priced.

These 'rollators' and trolleys can make a big difference to the person you care for's sense of security, comfort and convenience both inside and outside the house. They are lightweight and the dimensions are such that they can usually be easily used around the house. Some have a seat if the user needs to rest for a moment. Users can also sit and move about with their feet on some models (for example, while working in the kitchen) and they all fold up for convenient storage in the car boot or a cupboard. Some have a tray incorporated for carrying meals and drinks around the house;

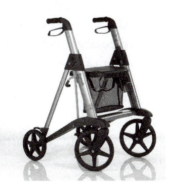

Figure 7: Stannah's active rollator, with basket

others have a basket (rather like a bicycle basket) so that packages, books, plants etc can be moved safely.

****

My mother was very obstinate about using a stick even though it was clear that she was very 'wobbly' on her feet. She would drag herself around the house clutching walls and doorframes. When she went out she would hang on to one of us. But when she spotted a three-wheel 'trolley' in a magazine small-ad she decided it was the very thing. And it was. She could use it inside and outside the house and it seemed to give her back a sense of independence.

****

For those who find walking even a short distance difficult or uncomfortable, there are many electrical scooters and power chairs available. Some of them are lightweight and will fit into the boot of a car. They are not a cheap option, but the cost may well be worth it to you and the person you care for.

Temporary support equipment

If your relative or friend requires temporary support equipment for getting around, the NHS is responsible for providing 'personal mobility aids'. For temporary walking aids, you will usually need a recommendation from a physiotherapist, who will advise on the right equipment. Referrals to physiotherapists can come through any of the following:
- local hospital
- community health service (district nurse)
- local health centre
- doctor (GP).

So, for example, if your relative or friend has been admitted to hospital with a fracture, then when s/he is discharged the hospital will ensure that the physiotherapy department measures for and provides the correct equipment to help her/him get around. If s/he has a fall at home and perhaps just needs some extra support to help her/him walk until fully recovered, then the best thing might be to ask about referral to a physiotherapist through the GP or district nurse.

The NHS provides mobility equipment on loan. It is not allowed to charge for equipment, but in some cases you or the person you care for may be asked to pay a returnable deposit to ensure return of the item. In some cases this system has been introduced because loaned crutches, for example, and other small items are frequently never returned to the hospital from which they have been borrowed.

Aids and equipment needed for long-term use may be obtained, after assessment by an occupational therapist (OT), from your local social services department. The OT will also be able to advise you about voluntary organisations and private companies that may also be able to help. For very temporary use (for example, during a holiday visit from a relative) the Red Cross provides a hire service.

Several companies manufacture mobility equipment. An OT from your local social services department may be able to give you advice about such companies and also voluntary organisations who may give grants towards equipment. But if you do not want to contact social services, most of these commercial companies advertise freely in magazines, newspapers and on the internet. Do not think that because they are commercial organisations these companies are selling inferior equipment. Most are reputable firms who rely on recommendation to retain custom and many have their own advisors to help you choose the right aid. Remember to specify to the seller if the person needing help has a disablity (s/he does not need to be registered disabled) and then s/he may be exempt from paying any VAT on equipment.

Getting upstairs

For some disabled and elderly people, getting upstairs is the only difficulty. They can walk around, carefully and slowly perhaps, and they are able to drive or use public transport as required. But for one reason or another they cannot climb stairs. Sometimes the problem is not the stair climb itself but the length of time it takes to negotiate the stairs. For example, if the only lavatory is upstairs, this may make considerable difficulties for someone with bladder problems or indeed for anyone on diuretics, which tend to create 'urge incontinence'. There are grants available to help disabled or infirm people to make adjustments and improvements to their home, which will allow them to continue living there. First port of call once again is your local library or local council website or enquiry service. For example, the disabled person you care for might be eligible for a grant to convert a downstairs room into a toilet or bathroom.

If the person you care for is totally unable to climb the stairs and a move to ground-floor accommodation is out of the question, then the classic answer is a stairlift. As with mobility aids, there are a number of firms which supply these and a grant may be available towards the cost. It is not widely known that many suppliers will renovate and supply second-hand stairlifts, which cuts the cost considerably for the buyer. You or the person you care for should be sure to ask about this when investigating a stairlift as not all companies will tell you this up front.

Before investing in the expense of a stairlift, it is worth your checking very carefully that the person concerned will be able to use it. Some mobility problems will mean that this is not an option. This also applies to anyone with early dementia, who may not be able to learn to use the stairlift properly.

Other factors

There are many very simple steps you can take to help the person you care for to be more generally mobile or to make the most of the mobility s/he has. Things like ensuring good lighting around the home, preventing clutter on stairs and in passageways, and installing extra handrails, may make a big difference to general ease and comfort. More details about these steps are to be found in Chapter 1, First steps.

In the 'Further useful information' for this chapter I have listed examples of suppliers of information and equipment to aid the disabled and elderly in getting about. To find out what transport schemes are available in your area, the best recommendation is to contact your local authority directly or ask for information in your local library.

Chapter 4

Problems with nutrition

My mother hated cooking even though she had brought up a large family and cooked good meals for us all. When he retired my father took over the cooking and it was something he really enjoyed. However, after he died Mum was faced with cooking again and didn't even have the satisfaction of cooking for others. She often said that she couldn't be bothered to make a meal. She used to go to the lunch club in the sheltered housing complex where she lived and we tried to make sure that she had enough high-quality food to prepare simple and quick snacks, sometimes using the microwave to speed things up. However, we couldn't entirely stop her filling up on sweets and chocolates, which she enjoyed, nor, to be honest, did we want to. As long as she kept well we thought we'd reached a 'happy medium'.

****

Generally, the nutritional requirements for the older age group are the same as for all adults, although there is a smaller energy requirement and very possibly an increase in the need for vitamin D, especially if an elderly person is housebound and therefore does not go outside much. But worry about malnutrition in their elderly relatives or friends is one of the most common concerns expressed by carers. Sometimes the concern is with becoming overweight. This tends to occur in the young elderly and needs to be addressed by encouraging more activity and keeping to a well-balanced diet. Activity tends to decline with age so less energy is expended. The energy requirement for a woman drops from 2200 kilocalories per day at the age of 18 to 1810 kilocalories at the age of 75. It is therefore important that the diet of an overweight elderly person is of a high quality and that so-called 'empty calories', obtained from sugar and starchy foods (refined carbohydrates), are kept low.

More often carers are concerned that their relative or friend is underweight or that her/his reserves of energy seem low or that s/he takes a long time to fight off minor infections and that these factors may point to inadequate nutrition.

There are various causes of malnutrition in the elderly. One is social isolation. Elderly people living alone may find it too much bother to cook or prepare meals for themselves. They may only eat what they consider gives the least trouble to prepare. It is common to find that tea and biscuits at frequent intervals take the place of a properly prepared full meal. They may frequently say that it doesn't seem worth the trouble of 'cooking for one'.

Another problem is provisioning. It can be difficult to find smaller portions of fresh food when shopping, particularly in supermarkets, which still tend to cater for the 'nuclear family'. Storing excess food is a problem unless there is ample refrigerator and/or freezer space and a good supply of sealable containers for dry goods. Planning and shopping to provide a varied diet may seem onerous. Elderly men in particular may have no idea of the importance of a well-balanced diet and even less idea of how to achieve this.

Elderly people who dislike cooking or who do not know how to cook may not prepare adequate meals. It is very easy to purchase instant 'snack' foods, which are filling and don't need any preparation, so that hunger is not a problem to them. The need for a balanced diet may not be obvious because the signs of malnutrition may be insidious and often take a long time to appear.

Elderly people in general may, through lack of stimulus, always eat the same things rather than keeping to a good mixed diet. They can get fixed in their ways and reluctant to try anything different. People in the early stages of dementia may continue to cook the same things over and over again because they are unable to look beyond what comes immediately to mind. Alternatively, people with dementia may forget how to prepare food or how to follow even a simple cooking sequence.

The senses of taste and smell do decrease with increasing age and this may mean that elderly people lose their ability to antici-pate and enjoy their food. Smoking and some drugs also affect these senses. Elderly people also secrete less saliva and they may suffer from a difficulty in swallowing (dysphagia). They may also have problems with teeth or dentures. All these physical problems may encourage them to neglect to feed themselves properly.

One thing to remember is that if the person you care for has a reduced appetite, then any food s/he eats should be of a high nutritional quality. Many people have become used to buying low-fat food items, including skimmed milk and fat-reduced cheese, because we are constantly told that these foods are 'better for your heart'. However, if someone is eating only very small amounts, then it is better to make sure that what s/he eats is packed with nutrients. Whole milk, full-fat cheese and eggs will be good foods where the appetite is small.

It is very easy for a carer to go for some time without realising that someone is not eating properly. For one thing, the person you care for might make an effort when you visit to have a meal available. S/he may fear your censure and lie about what s/he eats. S/he may not think it any of your business – after all, it is her/his life. Someone in the early stages of dementia may not remember whether s/he has eaten or not and may tell you that s/he has done so as part of the habit of 'confabulation' – filling in the gaps in her/his memory. As a carer you can help the person you look after to get the best from food in the ways I will now describe.

Learning to cook

Suggest or arrange cooking lessons if the person you care for has never been the main cook. Local authorities often have cookery classes which cater for the elderly or those living alone. Your local library will have details of these. But cooking lessons do not have to be formal. Any competent cook can show another person how to make a few simple dishes. This may be an area where younger members of the family who are too busy to assist with the main caring might be able to help. There are also many books available which cater specifically for people 'cooking for one', or focus on simple and quick-to-prepare meals. Some are available in large print (see Further useful information).

Shopping

Ensure enough food is available by making suitable arrangements for shopping. If the person you care for is able to shop alone you can help by discussing how to plan the shopping around her/his menus. People who haven't been in the habit of doing the food shopping need guidance, especially on 'store cupboard' items which they may previously have taken for granted as being available at home (think of salt, pepper and bottled sauces, for example). Help your relative or friend to make out the shopping list in advance. If you take her/him shopping yourself, then it is still a good idea to make a list in advance but you will also be able to help her/him shop systematically and to make suggestions about newer and simpler products.

If heavy shopping is a problem you can help to arrange home

delivery. Most big supermarkets will arrange delivery of the shopping that you have selected in the store. You can also shop online from several of the big supermarkets and have the goods delivered within a tight (usually two-hour) time slot. In small villages the local shops may have informal arrangements to deliver shopping to the elderly or incapacitated. You may have to ask as they may not advertise that they do this service.

Another useful possibility is the local milk delivery, if your neighbourhood still has one. Where these services survive, along with the milk, many roundspeople deliver items such as bread, fruit juice, eggs, potatoes, yoghurt and bottled water. These are staple and/or heavy items which can be delivered directly to the doorstep of the person you are caring for; this will cut down on the amount of shopping required.

****

My mother-in-law had always made her own (delicious) gravy using meat juices from the roast, flour and stock cubes. She complained that she couldn't be bothered to 'go to all that trouble' when just cooking for herself. Therefore she didn't cook meat very often. I introduced her to the various makes of 'gravy granules' which make instant gravy with boiling water. Eventually we found one she liked and she took pleasure in cooking hot meat meals again.

****

Food storage

Consider food storage arrangements. The refrigerator should be easy to access and keep clean. Most modern fridge/freezer arrangements house the freezer on the lower level and the fridge at hand height, but older single fridges can be quite low and you may find that your relative or friend neglects food items on the lower shelves because of difficulty in bending down. If it is a floor-standing model, you may be able to raise it to make it easier for the person concerned to see inside and to reach for items as required. Even if s/he has never previously owned one, many people will find a small freezer very useful. It cuts down on shopping trips and ensures that certain foods stay fresh for longer. For example, if the person you care for uses just a little milk every day, most of even the small-size cartons will be wasted, but small amounts can be frozen in very small containers and moved to the fridge as needed. You can buy very small freezers or combined fridge-freezers, where the freezing compartment is quite small.

It is also a good idea to check the arrangements for dry-food storage. The most accessible cupboards should be kept for foods that are used every day. You can now obtain plastic food containers that are easy to open and easy to wash and keep clean. If the person you are caring for has not previously had charge of the kitchen stores, show her/him how to rotate tinned and packet goods and make use of use-by dates. Some of these tips may seem obvious, but elderly people often get into a rut in their everyday living arrangements and something as small as encouraging them to rearrange the food storage cupboards may make their lives astonishingly easier.

Make sure that there is a small contingency store of tinned or packet food so that if bad weather prevents shopping, or if a carer is prevented from visiting for a couple of days, some food is available. Tinned meat stew or tinned fish, tinned potatoes and packets of crackers and digestive biscuits make good standby food. Tinned soup is often popular as it is easily heated up and is hot and comforting. You may periodically have to remind your relative or friend of the store and make sure that s/he can still prepare this sort of food easily. For example, progressive arthritis may make opening tins more and more difficult (see Chapter 1, First steps, for details of appliances and equipment which can help disabled people).

Chapter 4

Food preparation

Make sure food preparation is as easy as possible. Modern appliances are a great help. If buying new appliances, think about oven-timers, automatic ignition on gas cookers, and simple-to-use controls. Consider buying a microwave oven for the person concerned, even if s/he has not used one before. (Be aware though that it is unlikely that someone with dementia will be able to learn to use a new appliance.) They can be used to defrost food, such as bread which has been stored in the freezer, and can speed up the cooking of simple but filling items like jacket potatoes. If the person you care for has not previously used a microwave oven, look for one with simple, basic functions. (This will probably be cheaper too.) Encourage the person you care for to make full use of pre-packed salads, cook-chill dishes and complete 'ready meals'. These are now readily available from supermarkets and via mail order, and while you may generally shun them in favour of home cooking, they can provide an important way of getting someone living alone to eat sensibly.

****

The best thing we did for my father was to buy him a microwave oven. He could cook ready meals, 'bake' jacket potatoes which he ate with baked beans and cheese, heat up soup and defrost a loaf whenever he felt like 'fresh' bread. He always claimed to be unable to cook but enjoyed learning the microwave controls and later bought himself a bigger 'all-singing, all-dancing' model to experiment with.

****

Check the stores of food in the fridge and larder at regular intervals. Partially sighted people may not be able to read 'use-by' dates, and those who have lost some sense of smell may not recognise 'off' odours from food in the fridge.

Alternatives to self-catering

You could arrange for your relative or friend to attend a 'lunch club', or a day centre where a meal is provided, once or twice a week. Some elderly people find this a real boon since it means that they do not have to think about and prepare a main meal every day. Others complain about the standard of the food and prefer to manage for themselves. Although an arrangement like this does not solve all the meal preparation problems, it does mean that you can be sure the person you care for is getting a nutritionally balanced meal at regular intervals. If s/he lives in a sheltered housing complex, there is often an associated 'club' or social centre where (usually midday) meals are laid on. Users will have to pay for the meal, of course, but this will be offset by the smaller shopping bill. In addition, you and other members of the family, or friends, can take turns to invite her/him round for a meal.

Check the local provision of 'meals on wheels'. Some local councils still provide a cooked meal ready-to-eat for people who cannot cook for themselves. Other local councils provide cook-chill or frozen food in foil containers which have to be heated up by the person receiving them. The WRVS also provide meals-on-wheels in some areas – sometimes in conjunction with the local council. You can check the provision in your local area via the internet: www.gov.uk/meals-home.

A number of firms will deliver frozen meals (for reheating) on a weekly basis. Your relative or friend will need to have sufficient freezer storage to use these. Most providers allow the user to choose from a range of menus so tastes and different diets can be catered for. The meals are generally good value, but the person you care for will need to be able to use a cooking appliance to reheat them properly. For this reason, such options are not always practicable for someone with dementia beyond the early stages.

Dealing with loss of taste and smell

Some drugs may affect the senses of taste and smell so get your relative or friend to check with the GP if you think this may be the case. Otherwise, the best way to stimulate these senses is by encouraging the person you care for to plan, think and talk about food and the menus and dishes which s/he is going to prepare. If you are serving a meal to the person you care for, take extra care with the presentation. Large portions may put off someone with a small appetite. It is better to offer a smaller portion and second helpings if required. You can also enhance the flavour of dishes by using more seasoning or sugar than you normally would, using stronger-flavoured food, such as mature cheese, smoked fish and strong pickles, and offering extra sauces, both savoury and sweet.

Dealing with physical disability

Make sure that food preparation and consumption are as easy as possible by providing the person you care for with any specially adapted plates, cups or utensils that may be needed (see Chapter 1 on aids and appliances). Many 'convenience' foods, such as frozen vegetables, boil-in-the-bag rice, and tinned meat and fish, are easy to prepare and perfectly nutritious, and you could encourage their use as part of meal planning. Electric tin-openers and mixers and blenders may be useful.

Teeth and mouth problems

Poor teeth, or ill-fitting dentures, will obviously affect the ability to chew. If possible, you should encourage the person you care for to have proper dental care at regular intervals. There are dentists who specialise in care of the elderly or in treating reluctant patients, and one very good way to find such a dentist is via an internet search (see Further useful information). You can get help with transport problems which make trips to the dentist difficult (see Chapter 3, Getting about). Many older people find it difficult to clean their teeth effectively. An electric toothbrush can help significantly.

Dysphagia

'Dysphagia' means difficulty in swallowing. There are many causes of this problem. If the person you care for has had a stroke, or has some degenerative disease such as multiple sclerosis, then any swallowing problems are likely to be quickly recognised by the medical team looking after her/him. However, many elderly people do develop dysphagia slowly, due perhaps to decreased salivary secretion or some benign condition. If you realise that s/he is having a problem with swallowing, arrange for her/him to see the GP to exclude any serious or treatable condition. The doctor may refer you/the person you care for on to a 'swallowing team' attached to the local hospital, or to the community speech-and-language therapist. Otherwise, a physiotherapist may be able to help. Sometimes there is no treatment which is helpful and you have to help the person you care for by making eating, and swallowing pills, easier.

****

My mother-in-law had real difficulty in swallowing pills and frequently complained of 'something in the throat', but the doctor couldn't find anything wrong and suggested it was a nervous condition. We had to crush all her pills to a powder for her and we used to mix them with a teaspoon of honey. When she went into hospital they didn't realise that she couldn't swallow and nobody checked whether she took her pills. It was only when we found them hidden in her bedside locker that we realised she hadn't been taking them.

****

High-protein drinks can be useful occasionally, and semi-liquid foods like yoghurt, porridge and milk puddings might be easier to swallow than 'chunky' food. You can purée vegetables and mash potato to make them easier to eat, and you can purée fruit and make a 'smoothie'. You may be able to get liquid versions of some drugs instead of pills if you explain to your doctor that your cared-for has a problem swallowing. Otherwise, you can mix powdered pills with a spoonful of something like yoghurt, honey, or ice-cream. However, you should check first that this is appropriate. Some pills are specially coated and have to be swallowed whole.

Malnutrition

Clinically evident malnutrition is rare. A sub-clinical deficiency is much more likely, and most doctors would agree that it is not always easy to distinguish between the frailty caused by physiological changes in the elderly (loss of muscle tone, for example, and stiffness of movement) and the physical decline which accompanies mild malnutrition. The nutrients generally considered most likely to be deficient are: potassium, folate, vitamin B12, vitamin D, and vitamin C.

As a carer you should be alert and aware of certain indications which might suggest a need for dietary improvement. Specific signs of nutritional deficiency are:

- Weight loss and loss of energy – This may indicate that insufficient food is being eaten, or that food is not being absorbed properly. (However, see Chapter 7 on dementia)
- Excessive thirst, urinary infections, sunken eyes – Any of these may indicate inadequate fluid intake
- Weakness and tiredness, sore gums, slow healing of wounds – Any of these symptoms may indicate low vitamin C intake
- Fractures, bone pain – These may indicate low vitamin D intake, though osteoporosis should be considered first

- Anaemia, tiredness and/or an inflamed tongue – Either symptom may indicate low intake of folic acid
- Tiredness, headaches, brittle spoon-shaped nails, a sore tongue – Any, or all, of these may indicate insufficient iron in the diet.

Generalised signs that might suggest attention should be paid to the diet include:

- Weight loss, complaints of tiredness and weakness
- Dry lips, painful mouth, sores (similar to cold sores) on lips and around mouth
- Dry, unhealthy look to the skin, and/or sore skin
- Constipation
- Ravenous appetite when given a meal, indicating a possible neglect of preparing own meals.

If you suspect that symptoms are related to nutritional deficiency, be sure to mention it to the GP. A doctor may be looking for medical reasons for any symptoms and, unless s/he has regular experience in looking after the elderly, may not think about their nutritional status. You can ask for the person you care for to be referred to a dietician if you are really worried, but you can do many simple things yourself to help improve things.

****

We had a very nasty experience when arriving to visit my mother-in-law one day. She had had a severe nosebleed and been unable to clean up properly. The place was a thorough mess, but she didn't seem to have knocked her nose or done anything to cause the bleed. When we consulted the doctor he could find nothing wrong but suggested we look at her diet. It turned out that although she had been making meals she never cooked vegetables (too much trouble) or ate any fruit. We don't know if this was the cause of the nosebleed but we brought her some vitamin pills and made her take one each day and made sure that there was plenty of fruit juice open in the fridge for her to use.

****

How to help

1. Ensure the person you care for takes a daily multivitamin pill. There are many to choose from, but check to ensure that the one you choose includes a good dose of vitamin C.
2. Ensure that s/he drinks a daily glass of fruit juice (not fruit drink or squash). Good helpings of fresh fruit and vegetables would also be useful. From the vitamin and fibre point of view, fruit and vegetables are interchangeable so if s/he does not like vegetables (many elderly men profess to dislike them), then fruit would be a good substitute and vice versa. Sometimes advice about 'five a day' leaves out the fact that either fruit or vegetables are appropriate. The one advantage of fruit is that most fruits can be eaten without cooking. Of course, many vegetables can also be eaten raw, but elderly people may find them difficult to chew in the raw state. You could make sure that a bowl of fresh fruit is always available and regularly replenished. You could also make sure to include salad in the diet.
3. Suggest a 'nightcap' of hot milk or a milky drink such as cocoa. It is better if this is made with full-cream milk rather than from one of the 'instant' hot chocolate drinks because these are usually made with dried skimmed-milk. Whole milk is better for an underweight person.
4. If bad teeth, or ill-fitting dentures, or sore mouth, discourage the eating of fruit or vegetables, purée some and mix with ice-cream, or gravy in the case of vegetables, to be eaten with the next meal.
5. Suggest 'instant' porridge oats for breakfast, quickly

cooked in the microwave. Again, this will be better if made with milk or if milk is added.

6. Leave tasty sandwiches in the fridge prepared with fish (tinned is fine), cheese, or egg and salad. Sandwiches can be a good meal for someone living alone and because they need no preparation, the person you care for may eat more. Eggs are particularly good in the diet as they are easy to prepare, can be cooked in many different ways and are very nutritious. They are also tolerated well by those with a poor digestion for meat. It is a myth that they raise cholesterol levels in the blood.

7. Take the person you care for out for a meal occasionally. This may re-kindle her/his interest in food, and you will gain an insight into what foods s/he likes to eat.

8. Give supplement drinks in-between meals. They come in many flavours and are usually made with milk. They are obtainable in many supermarkets and in pharmacies. You should not have to go to a health-food store to get them. Check the labels as some have a much higher sugar content than others. Sometimes it may be possible to get them on prescription. Ask the district nurse about this. However, beware of using these supplements as meal replacements. They often rely on a high sugar content to be palatable.

9. If preparing food for someone who is underweight then you can 'fortify' some dishes. For example, you can add a couple of spoons of dried milk to yoghurt, cereals, custard and hot drinks (even when these have been made with milk). This will add extra protein. Dishes such as scrambled eggs can be made with cream instead of milk, and cream can be added to soups, sauces and many drinks. Butter should be used in preference to any 'spreads' and can be added to mashed potatoes (along with whole milk) or vegetable servings. Grated cheese can also be used to top mashed potatoes and vegetables.

10. Do not buy 'reduced fat' or 'light' versions of foods for the person who is underweight.

Special needs

In general, doctors recommend that a good varied diet provides all the nutrients a person needs, but any acute illness in the elderly may be accompanied by a loss of appetite and they may take longer to recover than younger people. Some maladies that are more common in older people, such as leg ulcers and pressure sores, take longer to heal if the diet is poor. If the person you care for suffers from an acute or chronic condition, then you might want to consider giving a food supplement. Vitamin C, zinc and the B vitamins are all easily available in pill form and you might consider adding these to your cared-for's daily diet. If s/he finds it difficult to take conventional pills these supplements can be found as easy-to-take 'chewable' jellied sweets or as a syrup. Be careful about excessive vitamin C. It will do no harm but may cause diarrhoea in high doses. If your relative or friend does not get out into the sun and open air much you might also like to consider suggesting s/he takes vitamin D, either in pill form or as cod-liver oil. It is better though, to encourage some time in the fresh air and sunlight.

Some literature on nutritional problems in old age and on dementia suggests that various traditional medicines may be useful. The most commonly mentioned are ginkgo (for memory problems and peripheral artery disease), ginseng (as a general pick-me-up), and glucosamine (for cartilage problems). Generally, none of these therapies will do any harm if your cared-for takes them in the recommended dosage, and they may do some good. However, ginkgo should be stopped well before the person you care for undergoes surgery as it can lead to haemorrhage. (For guidance on the safe use of traditional herbal medicines consult a good medical herbal guide (see Further useful information).)

Chapter 5

Social needs and keeping busy

Mum and I had always been very close and often shopped or had outings together. After Dad died, however, she seemed to rely on me entirely for all her entertainment and company, refusing to go out to the club she used to frequent or to accompany neighbours shopping as she had done before. I found it really difficult because I had my husband and children to look after as well, and there simply wasn't enough time in the day for all her 'demands'.

****

Elderly couples often come to rely on each other for company and entertainment and take up hobbies that they can enjoy together. Gradually old friends may die or move away and they may become isolated without even realising it. If one of the couple dies it may be a real shock to the survivor to discover that s/he has so few outside contacts. Many elderly parents turn to their children and younger family to fill the gap in their social life. This can put heavy demands on whoever is the main carer.

Another difficulty which sometimes arises is when previously physically fit elderly people become less fit and cannot socialise as they have been used to doing. Sometimes the physically fit member of the partnership dies first and the surviving elderly person finds difficulty in carrying on the social life which s/he enjoyed before, simply because there is no one to fetch things, drive her/him out, or help her/him to do what they previously did together. Again, the main carer may find s/he is under pressure to supply the missing help. This chapter examines the social needs of the elderly who are living alone and suggests ways in which these needs can be met by and shared amongst their carers.

Accept any help offered

After a bereavement it is natural for family to take extra care of the surviving relative, to give more time to her/him and to arrange activities which will please and distract – to try to 'fill the gap'. It is quite common for help offered by non-family, or those seen as 'outsiders', to be refused in the early days. The family may feel that the bereaved person can cope only with close relatives or friends and probably have the intention of asking for help after a short time has passed. However, help which is refused may not be offered again as those offering may feel rejected. It is also human nature for offers of help to come flooding in at times of crisis and to tail off as things seem to be getting back to normal. It is very important for the immediate family, and especially for the main carer, to encourage the person needing help to keep in touch with old friends and acquaintances and to take up any regular activities again.

If neighbours and friends offer help, therefore, do not turn it down. One very good solution is to ask them to do something specific – give a lift to the shops, have a shared meal or drop in for coffee once a week, for example. Or you could ask a neighbour to accompany the person you care for on her/his first visit back to a regular club or church. Do not be put off if your cared-for at first says that s/he would rather do these things with you. It is important for her/him to re-establish a wider social life and it is important for you to have alternative helpers to call on.

If help is not offered, remember to ask for it. Neighbours may hold back because they are afraid of interfering, or members of social clubs or groups may feel embarrassed and not wish to intrude. But many people welcome being approached and asked to help and are glad to feel that they can do something which is practical and useful.

Start with the immediate environment

When considering social needs and any changes which need to be made, start with the immediate environment. However often your relative or friend is taken out or visited, s/he has first to get used to the new condition of living alone and furthermore in an environment where reminders of her/his previous life and companionship are constant. You may spot small changes around the home which if made would really help her/him in daily life (see Chapter 1, First steps). However, don't suggest changes too soon after a bereavement as it may upset your relative or friend, who may like the comfort of still seeing her/his partner's chair in its regular position or dressing gown hanging behind the bedroom door. Things which will provide distraction and prevent too much morbid thinking will be useful. If a daily paper was not delivered before, then now might be the time to arrange this as it makes a useful routine to the beginning of the day. The daily postal delivery will probably be looked forward to much more than before and there are many ways to enhance this experience. Relatives who live too far away to visit can be encouraged to send letters and postcards regularly. A magazine subscription can give a regular lift in spirits and mail order catalogues, which may be seen as a nuisance to those of us leading busy lives outside, may be looked forward to with enjoyment by someone with time on their hands. The person you are caring for might like to join a book club and receive regular books in the mail, or perhaps to take up a pen friend with regular letters to look forward to.

You and the person you care for might like to consider daily pastimes and hobbies and how these can be enhanced. If s/he is a reader and used to making regular trips to the library, then this can be continued. If s/he is a non-driver and the library is at some distance, investigate whether there is a mobile library van which calls locally. This is an excellent service and usually operates even in quite remote areas. The mobile library carries a good selection of books and will take orders for borrowing, just like the main library. They will also stock large-print books. Your local library and your local county council will have details of mobile library services. Alternatively, perhaps you could arrange for a neighbour to take your cared-for to the library regularly. This would provide an outing and a chance for social contact as well as the pleasure of selecting books to read. An avid reader who is happy to use a computer would probably enjoy ordering books via the internet.

Many elderly people enjoy using an ebook reader or a tablet. Do not dismiss the idea of introducing an elderly person to computers and the internet. Personal computers and tablets these days are very user-friendly and you certainly do not have to be particularly technically minded to use them. Social networking sites, email, and particularly Skype (so that you can see and speak to grandchildren and other relatives), are popular with many older people. As suggested below, a teenage member of the family may really enjoy showing Grandma or Grandpa how to use a computer to best advantage.

****

After my mother died we used to order books for Dad via the internet. He began to get very interested in the way we did this and eventually invested some money in a laptop and internet connection, which my teenage son set up for him. It gave him a whole new lease of life and he spent hours on the web and even used some chat rooms! He also emailed the grandchildren frequently and got a lot of pleasure from their replies. On birthdays he even used to send 'E cards'.

****

Many elderly people enjoy both television and radio programmes. It may be that they have carried on for years using a particular model of radio or television because they have become used to it and have never considered updating their systems. Newer systems may offer a larger screen, easier controls, clearer sound and an improved enjoyment of the media. And don't forget that BBC iplayer and its equivalents mean the ability to watch programmes on a computer or tablet at a time of the individual's choosing.

If the person you care for enjoys music, encourage her/him to upgrade her/his music system and to use an MP3 player, or CDs still, both for ease of use and for the sound quality. CDs can also be borrowed from the library. DVD/Blu-Ray players offer a range of entertainment.

For all entertainment media, consider how best the equipment can be placed to make it easy to use, taking into account the lifestyle and abilities of the person you care for. For example, if an elderly person has difficulty bending down it may make sense to place the DVD/Blu-Ray machine on a table or shelf beside the TV rather than on the shelf which is often provided below the TV stand. If the person you care for particularly likes to listen to the radio in the early morning, then it may be more important to have the radio in the bedroom than in the main sitting room, or perhaps to have an additional radio. S/he may enjoy watching TV in bed and an easy-to-use remote control may be important here.

For those who have poor sight, consider talking books. There is now a vast range, and they can be obtained in most high-street stores and can be borrowed from the library. They are also a very useful present idea. Many newspapers and magazines can be purchased in a spoken form (see Further useful information) and arrangements can be made for these to be delivered regularly by post. Ebook readers have the great advantage that the print size can be altered at will. They are easy to learn to use, and downloading of books is very simple.

****

My mother was partially sighted and after she died I was left with a large collection of talking books which I felt were far too good to just throw away. By chance I heard of a lady who attended my church and who had developed an eye condition which prevented her from reading. I offered her the collection and she was delighted. But there was a knock-on effect. Someone else in the church hearing about this began to run a lending library of talking books and quite a number of people benefited. Some had books to pass on and some wanted to borrow. I always felt that my mother would have approved of her 'legacy'.

****

Plan a pattern to the day

For someone living alone, a set pattern to the day can be a great help. A daily pattern will also help someone in the early stages of dementia to remain orientated. Mention has already been made of the daily paper and the postal delivery. If a cleaner or a professional carer comes in, then the times which are arranged are also part of the day's pattern. You could usefully help the person you care for to plan radio programmes or TV viewing as part of this pattern and to incorporate exercise such as a short walk or even a stroll around the garden daily. Meals also break up the day. The main meal might be best taken in the middle of the day because this will be better for the digestion, especially if s/he goes to bed early. A midday meal is also the best arrangement if the person you care for uses meals-on-wheels or has a carer come in to cook the meal.

The preparation of meals and snacks can be a very pleasurable activity and a good opportunity to incorporate short visits. A neighbour might drop in regularly mid-morning for coffee, or you might arrange your daily visit to coincide with tea-time. Further tips on keeping up a good standard of nutrition and making simple meals can be found in

Chapter 4, Problems with nutrition. A weekly pattern which incorporates regular shopping trips, visits to social clubs or to church, or visits from family members, will also help the person you care for.

Activities and hobbies

Most of their social life for my parents centred around their local Wine Circle, which was a real social club with weekly meetings, visits and dinner parties. When my father died my mother continued as a member of the Wine Circle and kept up with all her friends there. When she moved nearer to me a couple of years later she did try to join the local Wine Circle but said that she didn't find it very welcoming. I was really sorry because so much of her social life had dropped away.

****

There are many ways the person you care for can keep up with old activities and hobbies, even if circumstances have changed. These days almost every activity can be indulged in via post, telephone or the internet. Some examples of how hobbies can be adapted follow.

Crafts – If your relative or friend likes crafts, kits can be obtained by post, as can sewing and knitting patterns and wool and materials. Magnifying apparatus will help even those whose sight is impaired to sew, knit or do other craftwork. Model-making kits can be obtained by mail and there are enthusiasts' clubs and websites which can be joined. Look for local 'knit and natter' groups which mean that knitting can become a sociable activity.

****

My mum found the wintertime with the short days and dark nights the greatest trial after Dad died. In the autumn she used to order small dolls and knitting wool and materials to dress them. She would work on the dolls' wardrobes all winter and in the spring give them away as presents to friends' children, her grandchildren or as raffle prizes and gifts at Sales of Work and so on. She also made many as Christmas presents.

****

Gardening – If your relative or friend is a keen gardener, you will find that nearly all garden centres cater for those with mobility problems, with ramps, wheelchairs and raised displays. Seeds and plants can be obtained by post. You can organise the garden to incorporate raised beds for those who have difficulty bending down or kneeling. Raised kneelers can be bought at garden centres and by mail order. Long-handled garden tools can also be bought. If the person you care for has poor sight, plan the garden to include highly scented plants, clear paths made from white paving stones or gravel, and well-defined borders. If s/he has poor hearing, external telephone bells and door bells can be arranged for those who spend considerable time in the garden. If s/he has an allotment which is too big for him or her to work, then many local councils will divide plots up into smaller sub-plots among two or three persons.

****

Gardening was Dad's reason to live really. He had a large plot and grew all sorts of vegetables for himself and the family. When he began to suffer from angina he hated the thought that he might have to give up the garden. He bought several plastic stools and arranged them at strategic points all around the plot. Whenever he needed to he could sit down for a few moments and he could also sit down to weed parts of the vegetable beds or to sow seeds etc. This simple solution allowed him to continue gardening right up until he died.

****

Following a sport – If the person you care for likes to follow sport, this is where TV and radio really come into their own. Virtually every sport is featured these days on TV and radio and if this is a favourite hobby there are magazines and papers catering for most sports and most of these can be obtained by a postal subscription or through the local newsagent, or increasingly to download onto a tablet or laptop. There are literally dozens of websites which are concerned with sport. Tickets for games can be bought by telephone, by post and online. Local sports clubs sometimes have special concessions for pensioners. A neighbour who has a similar interest might be delighted to watch a match with the person you care for.

****

My mother-in-law was a racing enthusiast and enjoyed a regular bet on the horses, which my father-in-law always used to place for her when he walked down to the betting shop. After he died we helped her to continue this interest by setting up a telephone betting account (she didn't feel able to manage online betting) for her and arranging satellite TV so that she could watch a dedicated racing channel whenever it took her fancy.

****

Cooking for one and for others – The person you are caring for may enjoy cooking but still feel it isn't worth spending time cooking for one. You could suggest shared meals with a neighbour or friend. Allow her/him to invite you and the family round for a meal rather than feeling that you must always invite them. Use bulk recipes to help her/him stock her/his, or your, freezer. Suggest making cakes for sales and fêtes. Find out about the local WI market shop or stall. Buy some of the many cookery books which specialise in cooking for one or pick up 'suggested meal' recipe cards from supermarkets when you shop. If your relative or friend is fit and mobile, s/he might like to attend (or teach at) specialist evening classes in such things as cake icing or speciality cookery.

Painting, art and design – If the person you care for enjoys painting or drawing or design, help her/him to set up a room, or part of a room, as a 'studio' with good lighting and all the required equipment. Artists' materials can all be obtained by mail order. You could help her/him to set up a website to sell her/his paintings or find out how to hold displays in local town centres and galleries. Paint, charcoals, paper and canvas all make good presents. S/he could join a local art club. Small local publications such as parish, school and college magazines, would welcome help from an accomplished artist or designer to arrange layout, incorporate pictures and so on.

Chess, bridge etc – If the person you care for enjoys card games or chess, there are nearly always local clubs which welcome new members for chess, bridge, whist and so on. These clubs often have an informal system of giving lifts to enable less able members to come to meetings. If your cared-for is housebound, s/he could perhaps host meetings. Chess and bridge can be and often are played by post and via the internet, and many newspapers have chess and bridge 'puzzles' for solution. Many games have national and international enthusiasts' clubs which often issue a magazine or newsletter.

****

My elderly aunt enjoyed card games of any description. Neighbours and friends sometimes popped round to spend the evening playing cards but her social life really took off when she suggested a regular 'card games' session at the local day centre she attended. The people who ran the centre were very helpful and enthusiastic and eventually a separate afternoon card session was arranged. There were two 'spin-off' clubs formed for different games and these started to meet in each others' houses.

****

Sharing the load

In many situations, one family member, friend or neighbour is the principal carer. It is easy for this principal carer to fall into the way of thinking that s/he has to cope with all the social needs of the person for whom s/he is caring. This can sometimes feel like an intolerable burden. However, even family members who live at a distance or who have heavy working schedules or young children to care for can help to lighten this burden and gain a sense of being useful to their relative. Relatives or friends who live at a distance can still keep in touch and provide regular entertainment by telephone calls, letters and small gifts sent by post. Letters are particularly welcomed by elderly people living alone. Family members or friends who work full time may nevertheless be able to organise mail order and web-based shopping, or may volunteer to pay for help and companionship for their relative. (It is possible to arrange for 'paid companionship'. See Chapter 9 on Care agencies.)

Family members and other friends with small children can have quite a vital part to play. There is often an affinity between young and old and if your elderly relative is reasonably fit and active, s/he may enjoy being asked to babysit occasionally. Otherwise, short visits are best if children are very young and it is useful to centre the visit around something – showing Granny the video of the nursery school play or taking a present of a special cake to share, for example. Your elderly relative or friend may really enjoy photos, recordings, and pictures and cards drawn by children, and most children enjoy creating things for the elderly. Someone with young children is also in an ideal position to suggest that schools and nursery schools invite the elderly to see school plays, concerts and shows and to receive harvest gifts and so on.

Teenage children tend to be rather self-centred and may not want to bother with their elderly relatives, but they can be encouraged to do shopping and small DIY jobs and many of them will be happy to purchase musical or computer equipment on your relative's behalf or to give advice on the best equipment to buy, or to set it up to ensure the best quality sound/picture etc.

****

After Dad died we wanted to ensure that Mum still felt loved and knew that we would all keep in touch. However, we agreed that in her case it would be a bad idea to arrange that one of us always called or visited on a particular day as, if these arrangements fell through, we knew she would be bitterly disappointed. Instead we all made sure to either phone or visit at least once a week. As there were four of us she had plenty of phone calls and visits but didn't start worrying about (for example), 'It's Tuesday and Sarah hasn't phoned yet'.

****

It sometimes seems that those we care for fall into one of two groups: those who love socialising and going out and who perhaps seem to make too many demands on the carer's time to fulfil this social need, and those who refuse to go out more than they have to and who pour cold water on any plan for outings and social events. If the person you care for is someone who enjoys socialising and is fit and able, then s/he is very likely to arrange her/his own social life. The problem that often occurs is that the person is unable to get out and about because of an inability to drive or some disabling physical condition. Then the carer may feel that s/he has to be frequently on call to provide transport or help with getting about. Chapter 3 on just this subject suggests many solutions to this problem. You should also make use of any lifts offered and of transport provided by local authorities. For example, many day centres arrange transport to enable their constituents to attend their events. To find out what is available, contact the individual day centre, ask at your local library or council office or use the internet to get information.

'Day Centre' is a generic term for places and organisations which provide services ranging from simple social 'clubs' with games, singsongs, bingo etc, to hot meals, chiropody, physiotherapy and day-long respite care. Some of these centres and clubs are run at community hospitals, some from care home premises and some at local church and community halls. Some are run by the care homes themselves as a 'halfway house' for possible future residents, some are run by local authorities, and some by local charities, churches and caring agencies. Each has a different character and it is worth trying several to find out which is best suited to the person you care for.

Do not spurn the idea of day care because you picture this as demeaning to your friend or relative. Most people who attend them enjoy the company and activities and for those with dementia, who become increasingly unable to entertain themselves, the day at the day centre provides both company and essential stimulation.

****

My friend wanted to organise visits to a day centre for her mother and asked for information at the local doctor's surgery. Unfortunately they didn't understand quite what she was asking. When she took her mother to the day centre they were both horrified as it seemed to cater mainly for old people with dementia. My friend's mother refused to go there again and unfortunately was put off ever trying another.

****

As well as providing entertainment and other services, such centres also enable those who attend to make new friends and may help to form the basis of an extended social life. However, neither you nor your relative/friend should feel that it is necessary to rely for a social life on clubs which cater exclusively for the elderly or disabled. Many charities welcome input from older people and most local branches of national 'interest' groups do not operate any age restriction.

If the elderly relative or friend for whom you provide care falls into the 'antisocial' category you may find yourself desperately seeking ways of providing entertainment and fulfilling her/his social needs. Sometimes there is a physical reason behind an apparent lack of interest in outings or visitors. For example, someone suffering from urge incontinence (needing to get to a toilet in a hurry) may not be able to contemplate going out to a place where toilets are not close at hand. Then again, someone in the early stages of dementia might be actually afraid of leaving familiar surroundings.

If you are unable to establish a physical reason, you may be able to take a step-by-step approach. For example, you could suggest and encourage a short walk, followed by a trip to the local shops followed by a longer shopping expedition. Or you could arrange for a neighbour to drop by whilst you are there and then come again and stay for a few more minutes on a subsequent date, leading on perhaps to longer visits. However, it is important to remember that, whatever our opinion may be about what would 'do them good' or 'cheer them up', our relatives and friends are independent people and their likes and dislikes are part of what they are. It is not the responsibility of the carer to ensure that they are entertained or forced into activity which they may not like or appreciate. If the person you care for refuses to go out or to accept offers of entertainment it is ultimately her/his choice and responsibility. It doesn't mean that you have to fill the gap by spending more time with her/him than you can comfortably manage.

Chapter 6

Recognising medical conditions – including dealing with accidents and admission to hospital

I visited Mum every day. One day calling round after work, I found her sitting in front of the TV as usual but she was confused and unable to talk properly. I thought at first that she had had a fall and hit her head and I called the doctor. He explained to me that in fact Mum had had a tiny stroke. I had always thought that if you had a stroke you lost consciousness at the time and as a result of the stroke lost the use of one side of your body. The doctor explained that a small stroke might just result in a feeling like 'pins and needles' in your arm and leg, for example.

****

As the carer and, possibly, chief person in the life of your elderly relative or friend, it is likely that you will be the one who comes into contact with her/him most often. There are some medical conditions which may affect the elderly in particular. They may not happen suddenly, their onset may be insidious, but the sooner they are recognised and treated the better. If your relative is not seeing a doctor regularly the symptoms may be missed. This section is not supposed to replace qualified medical help and advice but only to enable you as the carer to feel more able to make the decision to call for the doctor when required.

I have also included in this section a brief description of some of the minor medical problems to which the elderly are prone, with some tips on how to relieve them. In addition, I look at coping with accidents and emergency admission to hospital. I will start by looking at how to recognise:

- Dementia (page 81)
- Stroke (page 86)
- Diabetes (page 88)
- Heart attack and heart failure (pages 89 to 90)
- Concussion (page 92)
- Nutritional problems (page 92).

Dementia

Conventional medical textbooks are not always helpful when describing dementia. They generally mention that it begins with forgetfulness and describe its cause, but for the layman carer this is not enough. We have to recognise that elderly people are often forgetful, awkward, slow and obstinate. This does not mean that they are suffering from dementia. It is also difficult to admit to oneself that a loved one is becoming demented even if all the signs are obvious to others.

There are many types of dementia, but Alzheimer's disease is the one most people have heard of and it accounts for approximately 60 per cent of cases. Vascular dementia accounts for about 15 to 20 per cent. Some medical opinion considers that the line between vascular dementia and Alzheimer's disease is not really clear cut and it is becoming more common to see a diagnosis of 'mixed dementia'. Dementia can also result from a number of other, much more rare diseases and conditions, and a dementia-like condition can result from certain nutritional deficiencies (see Chapter 4, Problems with nutrition). If the person you care for has been diagnosed with one of the other primary causes of dementia, such as Huntington's disease, then it is likely you are already well aware of what this means. This section is aimed only at helping the carer to recognise the development of *previously undiagnosed* dementia. Some medical conditions and some infections (such as a urinary tract infection) can have symptoms similar to those of dementia, which is one reason why a medical diagnosis is essential if you suspect dementia in your relative or friend.

Dementia is progressive and gets worse over time. Symptoms are mild in the early stages and the carer can do a lot to help. Although some medical textbooks identify specific stages, particularly in Alzheimer's disease, these stages are not always present or recognisable to the untrained eye. Basically, the deterioration in Alzheimer's disease is gradual and insidious, whereas in the case of vascular (sometimes called multi-infarct) dementia the decline can be more step-like. Vascular dementia may be more easily recognised by the carer because you can observe immediate deterioration at each 'step' or minor stroke. Alzheimer's disease may go unrecognised for a long time if you are in constant daily contact with the person suffering.

As noted in Chapter 10, many people with dementia are supported by their partners in such a way that the dementia is disguised, or at least not recognised by even close relatives until some crisis (a death, accident or serious illness) leaves the sufferer temporarily unsupported. Here are some pointers which might make you suspect dementia in your elderly relative or friend.

Memory loss

Memory loss is more than just the 'forgetfulness' of old age. Look out for blank denials of events. 'No, my daughter didn't come yesterday'; 'I had no breakfast this morning'; even when you know that these events have happened. The person you care for is not being difficult. S/he really believes that these things have not occurred because the memory of them is lost. In the early stages of dementia, people can sometimes recall events after a few gentle reminders. 'Yes, your daughter came and brought those flowers, remember.' The pattern varies, and most people with dementia recall long-ago events more easily than recent ones, or can be prompted to remember by looking at photos, for example.

Sometimes people are aware of their memory loss and try to cover it up by 'filling in' the blanks. This can be very upsetting for the carer unless s/he realises what is happening. 'My purse is gone – the nurse has stolen it' probably means simply that the purse was put down and forgotten about. But never ignore a claim like this.

Difficulty in recognising time and dates

Difficulty in recognizing time and dates is often a fairly early sign. Your relative or friend may prepare a meal for expected visitors on the wrong day, for example. S/he may insist that it is Saturday when it is Wednesday. Even if you point out the date (in a newspaper, for example) it may make no difference. Another sign is doing things at an inappropriate time. S/he may telephone you in the middle of the night and not accept that it is night-time when you point this out. S/he may get up and dress at 10 pm or go to bed at midday. Very often people can still read the time if you point at the clock; it is just that it doesn't seem to mean anything to them. At first your relative/friend may only mix dates and times occasionally.

Neglecting personal care

Neglecting personal care is a very upsetting sign for most carers. Even formerly very fastidious people may neglect hygiene matters when suffering from dementia. At first the person you care for may make excuses – 'It isn't good to put too much soap on your skin'; 'I only wear this jumper for housework – it doesn't need washing'; 'I'm too tired to wash my hair today'. Later s/he may not even respond when you point out dirty clothes or a lack of washing and bathing.

Many people with dementia will passively allow themselves to be washed and dressed, although they will not initiate the actions. Others, especially in the early stages, vigorously resist any attempts others may make to assist with personal care.

Refusal to recognise the needs of others

Refusal to recognize the needs of others may alert you at an early stage. The wife who, when her husband is ill, continually complains because he doesn't take her out; the husband who demands that his wife cook a hot meal when she is unable to see to do so – these are examples of what appears to be selfishness. Carers should be alert if this is not the norm for their elderly relative or friend.

Fears and delusions

It is not unusual for people with dementia to suffer delusions. They can also sometimes be highly suspicious and believe that others are trying to harm them or to persecute them. They may become excessively frightened. An elderly lady who has always been sensibly security conscious in the past may suddenly start to pile furniture in front of the door in case someone breaks in, or may refuse to let the carer into the house 'because she is trying to kill me.' Your relative/friend may tell you that someone s/he knows dropped in for tea the day before when you know for a fact this is not true.

Rambling speech or inability to follow conversation

Someone suffering from dementia may not be able to explain something in a way that makes sense to you, even though s/he is able to talk and is really trying to explain.

'It was terrible…..it just rang and rang……I didn't believe it.' (Someone came to the door and rang the bell several times.) It may take several attempts for you to understand and s/he may just give up the effort if you press too hard. On the other hand, s/he may be able to carry on a simple conversation, but if you make a suggestion, 'Shall we go into the garden,' s/he may answer at random or refuse your suggestion because s/he just cannot make sense of it.

Inability to initiate actions

Often people with dementia find it hard to begin an action. For example, you may place a cup of tea by their side but unless you say 'Drink your tea now,' they may just ignore it. Someone who is living alone and who has this problem may never take themselves to bed of their own volition, or alternatively may not get up and dress without someone to prompt them.

Wandering/walking about seemingly without purpose

Many of us are familiar with the idea of the old person who 'wanders the streets', and this is a great worry for carers. As a rule, those with dementia appear to be either wanderers or not. There doesn't seem to the observer to be any reasoning behind the wandering, although it is thought that there is always a purpose behind the apparently aimless walking. On occasion, someone may be able to explain that the person was going to the shops or 'looking for so-and-so'. But often if you try to ask where someone was going, s/he may be unable to explain properly.

****

For some time we put my mother's symptoms down to other things – she was depressed following Dad's death; she needed company; old people often become frightened and confused. After all, she always offered us a cup of tea when we visited and smiled and nodded in the right places. But it was a façade. Her innate social skills were masking the fact that she could not make sense of our conversation and that, although she could follow the ritual for making a cup of tea, she couldn't initiate other actions alone.

****

Stroke

Many of us associate a stroke with a vision of someone turning purple in the face and collapsing unconscious, 'having an apoplexy' as the old books would describe it. In fact a stroke may be so mild that it goes almost unnoticed.

There are two kinds. Put simply, one is caused by a 'bleed' in the brain and this type of stroke may come on gradually. The person affected may complain of an intense headache, which is not relieved by normal painkillers; s/he may start to move very slowly, to slur her/his words and to be unable to understand what you say to her/him. S/he may vomit.

The second type of stroke is caused by a blood clot which prevents blood reaching a part of the brain. This is likely to be more sudden in onset. The sufferer may stop moving or speaking suddenly; s/he may fall down; her/his face may distort downwards on one side; s/he may lose the use of the arm and leg on one side; s/he may lose consciousness.

If the person you are caring for showed any of these signs it is likely that you as the carer would call the doctor immediately. A less easily recognised stroke might be so mild that the sufferer simply admits to feeling tired or dizzy; s/he may say that an arm or leg feels heavy or that there is from tingling or 'pins and needles' in the limb.

****

My dad complained of a headache for several days, although he refused to go to the doctor. Then one day he found that the words in the newspaper made no sense to him. He slept for several hours and woke feeling slightly better. The headache gradually passed off and he was able to read again. But he had to re-teach himself some things previously taken for granted, like how to tune the video recorder. In our ignorance we were just glad that he was feeling better. In fact, when he saw the doctor for something else months later the doctor said he had probably had a stroke caused by a 'bleed' and that he was lucky to have recovered as he had.

****

Subtle signs to be alert for are:
- Difficulty speaking
- Complaints of heavy or tingling limbs on one side of the body
- Inability to use an arm or leg in the usual way. (For example, when presented with a meal the person may use just one hand and a fork when normally s/he would handle a knife and fork in the traditional manner)
- Drooping of one side of the face
- Sudden inability to make sense of printed words or of the spoken word
- Headache which is not relieved by normal painkillers
- Loss of balance.

People who suffer a mild stroke may recover completely in a few hours, or days, or they may retain a minor impairment. Where multiple strokes happen, any impairment may get worse and remain worse with each stroke (see: Vascular dementia, page 79). However, there is no set pattern to strokes and someone may make a very good recovery from a second stroke after making only a slow recovery from the first one.

If you suspect even a mild stroke, it is essential to call the doctor. Prompt treatment is known to improve the chances of recovery.

Diabetes

If the person you care for is a diagnosed diabetic, you and s/he will know the treatment (tablets or injections) which has to be taken and the signs which indicate a need to call the doctor. However, in some older people, diabetes comes on gradually and it is useful to recognise the signs. In diabetes, the body is unable to store all the sugar derived from the carbohydrates eaten in a normal diet. The excess sugar remains in the blood and passes into the urine, carrying water with it. Signs to watch for are:

- Excessive thirst: this can be a misleading sign. Some elderly people living alone forget to make themselves meals and may neglect to drink enough. Your visit may trigger a realisation that they are thirsty and they may appear to drink excessively simply because they have become dehydrated due to self-neglect. This is still an important feature which needs addressing by you but it is not a sign of diabetes in itself. A diabetic, however, might, for example, drink two large tumblers of water or squash and still not appear satisfied, perhaps wanting another couple of glasses 15 minutes later.

- With the excessive thirst goes frequent passing of large quantities of urine. However, many elderly people need to use the toilet more often simply because bladders get weaker with age. In addition, if the person concerned is taking a diuretic, s/he will often pass water frequently – usually several times within a couple of hours of taking the dose. These frequent visits to the toilet are not signs of diabetes.

- Tiredness and weakness: again, it is important to remember that an elderly person may be more tired or feel less well than when they were younger and this is normal.

- Weight loss: however, type 2 or 'mature onset' diabetes usually occurs in people who are overweight and weight loss is unusual in this type of diabetes.

- Infections in the skin, such as boils or abscesses or thrush, and sore feet and legs may indicate diabetes.
- Blurred vision can sometimes occur.

As indicated above, none of these signs is an indicator of diabetes in itself, but two or three of these signs together should suggest that medical diagnosis is required. Treatment for elderly diabetics will usually consist of attention to diet together with tablets. Diabetes is a serious condition which can lead to other health problems. It should not be ignored or treated lightly, and if you suspect the person you care for may have diabetes you should arrange for her/him to see a doctor promptly. Uncontrolled diabetes is also a high risk factor for the development of dementia.

Heart attacks

A heart attack occurs when the blood supply to the heart is interrupted. A major heart attack is usually unmistakeable, causing severe chest pain, perhaps radiating to the arm and jaw; a feeling of pressure; pallor, or blueness, of the skin; and collapse. However, a minor heart attack, when the blood supply to only a small part of the heart is cut off, may produce much milder signs. Some elderly people may suffer from angina pectoris, when pain in the chest comes on following undue exertion and is relieved by rest. Angina is also sometimes triggered by a large meal and may be put down to indigestion, or it can be triggered by going out on a very cold day. The pain of angina varies according to the person, but it will almost certainly cause the person you care for to pause, to be unable to speak whilst in pain and to turn pale during the attack, perhaps breaking out in a cold sweat. Angina is treatable and if you suspect it in your cared-for you should ask for a doctor's appointment without delay.

In a mild heart attack the pain is often similar to an attack of angina and there may be slight nausea with shortness of breath, pallor and a cold sweat. The symptoms may pass within minutes, or hours, leaving the person you care for tired and shocked.

Because the signs of angina and a mild heart attack may pass quickly, they may be easy to ignore or to pass off as the signs of 'old age'. If you witness an attack and question the person you care for, you may find on enquiring that s/he has had several episodes which s/he has ignored or not mentioned to you.

****

Whilst living alone my father suffered what we later discovered was a heart attack one night and spent the night lying on the sofa waiting for morning before venturing to call the doctor. He later explained that the symptoms came and went at intervals but because they kept passing off and because it was night he 'didn't want to bother the doctor'.

****

Heart failure

Congestive heart failure occurs when the heart is unable to perform its usual functions adequately. This section will discuss gradual heart failure because sudden and acute heart failure has symptoms which would immediately prompt a call for medical assistance.

In gradual heart failure there is a reduced supply of blood to the tissues and to the lungs. Because the onset is gradual, at first the body is able to compensate. When compensation is no longer adequate, fluid begins to accumulate in the lower part of the body and in the lungs. The ankles and lower legs may swell, and at first this may only happen after a long day 'on the feet' or in the afternoons. Later on, the swelling does not go away even after a night of bed rest. The sufferer may get tired more easily and be unable to walk as far as before. S/he may also get breathless on exertion. S/he may need to sleep sitting up to breathe more easily. In the late stages, the abdomen may swell, and perhaps the hands, and you may notice a blue tinge to the lips, ears and fingernails. In advanced stages, the sufferer may be confused and lethargic and may not be able to respond quickly enough to signals to empty the bladder or bowels.

Signs to be alert for are:

- Swollen ankles and lower legs – on more than just the odd occasion
- Lethargy
- Breathlessness
- Needing to sleep sitting up in order to breathe easily.

Heart failure is treatable in its early stages and the person you care for should see a doctor if s/he has any of the above symptoms.

****

My mother's heart failure came on gradually, and because the pills she was prescribed caused her to vomit she stopped taking them and then consistently refused to see a doctor. My father was quite ill himself and unable to reason with her. Nor could we persuade her, although we were desperately worried. It was only when the district nurse called on a routine visit that the doctor was summoned. He explained that the dosage of the drug had to be carefully worked out by 'trial and error' and that a 'too high' dose was causing the vomiting. He gave Mum a reduced dose of her medication and she recovered and lived for several more years. However, after that we made sure that someone always went with her on visits to the doctor to listen carefully to instructions about any medication.

****

Concussion

Elderly people are more prone to fall over, even inside the house. A fall which involves a bang on the head may lead to concussion. Someone living alone who has a fall of this sort is very likely to be unaware that s/he is concussed. You may find that your elderly relative or friend is confused and suffering from a loss of memory of events just before and just after the incident which caused the concussion. If you discover her/him lying unconscious you would naturally call the doctor immediately. However, there is also the possibility that you will be the first visitor after a fall from which s/he has apparently recovered and of which s/he has no memory.

Signs to look for are:
- General confusion
- Slurred and confused speech
- Stumbling movement and imbalance
- Loss of memory
- Visible injury to the head
- Injury to other parts of the body indicative of a fall
- Vomiting and pallor of the skin.

If you suspect concussion, put the person you care for to bed in a darkened room and call the doctor. If you suspect any serious head injury, it is better to call an ambulance straightaway.

Nutritional problems

Nutritional problems may be an issue, particularly if your elderly relative or friend lives alone. Those living alone may find it too much bother to cook or prepare meals for themselves. They may only eat what they consider gives the least trouble to prepare – say, a cup of tea and biscuits at frequent intervals rather than a full meal. Or they may, through lack of stimulus, always eat the same things rather than keeping to a good mixed diet. They may also have lost some of the senses of taste and smell, which will mean that they no longer enjoy eating well. Chapter 4 is devoted to problems with nutrition (page 49).

Other common medical problems

Dad was living alone and seemed to be coping quite well, although it was clear that he wasn't particularly active during the day. For several days he complained of backache and, thinking it was just a result of sitting around too much, we tried to encourage him to get up and walk around more and gave him some standard painkillers. Then one day when my sister was helping him to change his clothes she discovered a nasty sore on his lower back. In fact it was a pressure sore and we had to call in the district nurse to have it dressed and treated. We were told it was caused by him sitting in one position and in the same chair for much of the day.

****

Pressure sores

Pressure sores used to be called 'bed sores', but they do not occur only when someone is bedridden. They are very painful areas of broken skin which form over bony parts of the body when the skin is pressed against bedding or furniture (a chair cushion, for example). They are more likely to happen in elderly people who are incontinent and who perhaps sit for some time in wet clothing as a result. They are also more likely to occur in people who do not move around much and spend time sitting or lying in one position. You should suspect a pressure sore if the person you care for complains of pain in any one area especially. Pressure sores are painful and need regular dressing from the district nurse. Prevention involves encouraging the sufferer to move around more, to change position frequently when sitting or lying down (you could encourage using different chairs to sit in at different times), to change their clothes when wet and to keep their skin clean.

Swollen feet and legs

Swollen feet and legs are not always a sign of anything serious. This swelling can occur as a result of sitting still too long in the elderly if their circulation is poor. Encourage the person you care for to keep mobile even if only around the house and suggest that when s/he sits, s/he puts her/his feet up. Relaxing/reclining chairs are very useful to encourage this.

Painful feet

Older people, particularly if they have trouble bending, may neglect their feet. This may result in long horny toenails, sores on the feet from shoes which rub, and an accumulation of hard skin. It is a good idea for any carer to help wash the feet at least once a week so as to spot trouble arising. Chiropody is available free to elderly people who have a medical condition, such as diabetes, and ought to be obtainable in their own home. Many types of comfortable slippers and shoes are now available by mail order aimed especially at the elderly and those with foot troubles.

Painful movement

Many elderly people suffer from painful movement to some degree through stiffness or through osteoarthritis and rheumatoid arthritis. Encouraging the person you care for to move around as much as s/he is able is a good thing to do. There are many over-the-counter painkillers available for minor aches and pains, but some elderly people need encouragement to take medication. For more severe pain, the doctor can prescribe more efficacious medication but you may still have the problem of compliance. There are several 'memory jogger' pillbox devices which you can buy, or you can try making the taking of pills part of the before or after mealtime routine.

Dealing with accidents

Prevention

An elderly lady lived down our street a few doors away from us. We used to see her out and about and knew her well enough to pass the time of day. Coming back from shopping one day I noticed an ambulance outside and my next-door neighbour told me that she had noticed the curtains had not been opened that morning and notified the police. Apparently the old lady had fallen and broken her hip. I was rather ashamed that I had walked by earlier and not even noticed the unopened curtains.

****

Before considering how to deal with accidents it is worth mentioning again how to prevent them. Lighting is very important. Replace lightbulbs promptly and use the highest wattage that the light shade and fitting allow (in this respect eco-bulbs which take a long while to warm up and give acceptable light are perhaps not appropriate). Consider free-standing or wall-mounted spotlights near to chairs used for sitting to read, knit etc. Make sure that stair lights can be switched on and off both at the top and at the bottom of the stairs and that halls and passageways are very well lit. A light-coloured paint or paper on the walls helps to make the most of the light. Kitchens may need extra 'spot' lighting around food preparation areas and bathrooms near mirrors.

Stairs and hallways need to be kept clear of clutter as much as possible, and pale floor coverings help to expose obstacles. A second handrail can be fitted to most staircases if required. Small rugs should either be taken up or backed with non-slip matting or backing. Loose edges to carpets should be fixed firmly down.

Grab rails can be fitted quite easily by someone reasonably competent in DIY. These are very useful in the bathroom and around front and back entrances, especially if there are any steps to be negotiated. If the person you care for is very shaky on her/ his feet, you might consider a guide rail from sitting room and bedroom to bathroom so that support is available on common routes inside the house. If the person you care for suffers from frequent falls, you should ask for a referral to the local 'Falls Team' (the GP will arrange this), who will visit and advise on ways to keep mobile, and on the correct walking aids. Leaflets on balance and preventing falls are also available from GP surgeries, Age UK and local council information points and websites.

Calling for help

Alarm-call systems can be very useful for your peace of mind. These usually work from a central unit placed at a convenient spot in the house. This unit connects to a telephone line with a microphone so that should the person you care for press the contact button, someone from the call surveillance centre will answer to offer help or reassurance, or to contact you or an alternative named contact. Usually there is also a wrist- or neck-pendant with a call button which the person concerned is supposed to wear at all times during the day. The idea behind these alarm-call systems is excellent. Unfortunately, the system does ask for some measure of compliance from the user and this may be where a problem arises. Many elderly people simply object to wearing the pendant/bracelet, perhaps because it makes them feel 'old' or because they feel that they do not really need it.

****

My friend arranged an alarm-call system for her elderly mother because she was worried in case she might fall and be unable to reach the telephone. Her mother appeared to accept the idea and agreed to pay for it and oversaw its installation quite happily. The only thing was, she would never wear the pendant. Whenever my friend went round she would find it lying on a table or a kitchen counter. Her mother said that she always had it nearby but of course if she had fallen she might not have been able to reach it.

****

Another problem arises if your relative/friend is in the early stages of dementia. S/he may switch the control box off, or unplug it because s/he has grown used to unplugging electrical items when not in use, or simply because s/he forgets what it is there for. If the power is cut off, the control centre will normally try to contact the 'named contact' – probably you – and you may find yourself frequently called out at all hours just because the system has been switched off.

****

Once when we called round we found that a tablecloth had been wrapped around the call unit. After a lot of questioning we worked out that Mother-in-law had pressed the button by mistake and been frightened by the 'disembodied' voice which asked if she was all right. The person at the control centre had tried to tell her how to switch the thing off but she had not understood and had tried to muffle the sound instead.

****

Many designs of telephone now come with 'one-press' buttons which can be programmed to call a particular number. These can be very useful for the person you care for as you can set them up to dial your number, an alternative number and perhaps the emergency services at one touch. This is a great aid to someone who has poor sight, poor co-ordination or some confusion. You can also obtain telephones with larger-than-normal push buttons for those with poor sight or stiff fingers. There are some reasonably cheap models of mobile phones which offer one-touch dialling and a 'panic button' on the back which will dial pre-set numbers in succession until a response is reached.

If possible, ask the nearest neighbours to keep an eye on the house of the person you care for and alert you if they see signs of trouble – undrawn curtains, lights on all night, milk or newspaper not taken in. Some neighbours might be prepared to hold a key, but you should be careful that both you and the person you care for are happy about this. In some country areas the local milk delivery person or the postman/woman will keep an eye out for elderly householders.

Keep a good, well-stocked first-aid kit on hand in the house of the person you care for in case of accidents. You might also consider going on a First-aid/First-response course in case you discover her/him after an accident and have to wait a while for an ambulance. In some country areas where there might be a long wait for an ambulance even after the emergency services have been called, local volunteers provide a 'First-response' service where a trained person comes to the house and initiates resuscitation techniques or first-aid procedures whilst you wait for the ambulance. Various groups, including some Women's Institutes and The St John Ambulance, organise this scheme.

It might also be worth keeping a packed 'emergency night bag' or case ready in the house and letting neighbours and friends know where it is, or leaving a prominent note of its whereabouts. If the person you are caring for does have an accident and is taken to hospital in your absence, then there need be no panic about packing nightwear and toilet things for the hospital.

In 'A&E'

If the worst happens, and the person you care for has a fall, or an accident, and the ambulance is called, s/he will be taken to the nearest hospital with an Accident and Emergency (A&E) unit and this is where s/he will wait to be assessed. Most A&E units now operate a 'triage' system. People arriving at the unit will be seen by a senior and specially trained nurse who will assess how quickly they need to be seen by a doctor. If you are with the person you care for you will find that the length of time you have to wait will depend on many things, including the seriousness of any injury, the number of other more serious cases awaiting attention, the time of day and the day of the week. Sunday night is still traditionally the worst day/time on which to have an accident requiring care in A&E. While waiting you should not allow the person you care for to eat or drink unless the nursing staff have told you that you may do so as this may interfere with any anaesthetic required.

Waiting in A&E can be very traumatic. Hospitals differ in both their level of care and their efficiency, but the most common complaint from those waiting is of a lack of information. Although the unit looks busy and is crowded with people in uniform of various kinds, it may seem a daunting task just to find out what is happening in your individual case. Many units have no obvious central information desk, and there appears to be no one to ask what is happening. It is worth remembering that A&E departments have performance 'targets' which they are supposed to maintain in terms of waiting time for patients and treatment. You may not want to appear to be the one 'making a fuss', but once again, persistence generally pays off in terms of getting attention. Keep asking and don't be afraid to be assertive. But don't confuse assertiveness with aggression. Most hospitals have very strong 'non-aggression' policies and they are rightly concerned about any form of anger or violence shown to staff.

****

My mother-in-law was taken to hospital following a fall. They suspected that she had a broken hip. She was taken to A&E at 10 am and they began a series of tests and X-rays. My husband and son took it in turns to wait in A&E with her. At 6 pm the hospital told them to go home as she was about to be admitted and to telephone within the hour to find out which ward she would be on. When I telephoned at 9 pm I was horrified to find that she was still waiting in A&E. We went back to the hospital to be with her, but still she did not get admitted to the Elderly Care ward until after midnight.

****

Some hospitals now have a ward where people are admitted temporarily. It may be called the 'Medical assessment unit' or the 'Short stay ward' and it is usually close to the A&E department. The person you care for may be admitted here if the results of tests and X-rays taken in A&E do not define the underlying problem but the staff at the hospital feel that they should not be sent home immediately.

In hospital

If the person you care for is admitted to the Elderly Care department (you may still think of it under the old term 'Geriatric Care') do not be alarmed. Times have changed and Elderly Care wards are now better staffed and better organised generally than they were in the past. Much of the basic 'hands-on' care of patients is now carried out by healthcare assistants (they may have another title depending on the hospital) who have more time to give than the nurses do, and most of these are well trained and enjoy working with elderly people. These are the staff who will help elderly patients to wash and dress, who will make them comfortable, chat to them and if necessary help them with meals etc. It is worth your getting to know them. You will also find that careful records are kept, not only of medicines and treatment given but of individual care. For example, the care assistants will note that they have washed or helped a patient to shower or washed their hair and so on. Notes about this care are usually kept in a folder near the bed and when you visit you can read these notes and ask any questions about the care or medication your relative/friend has received.

There will also usually be a leaflet or folder which gives details of the facilities available at the hospital and of any extra help that you need to provide – for example, in terms of taking away clothing and nightclothes to be washed and returned. It is worth trying to arrange for a member of the family to visit every day, not only to cheer your cared-for but also to keep in careful touch with the level of care provided. If the person you care for is suffering from dementia and any assessment is to be made by a specialist, you can ask to be present and you should definitely make a point of talking to the doctor in charge of the case. The doctor's name will usually be displayed on a sign somewhere near the bed, or on a ward plan which is available for you to see. Remember that elderly people, even if they are mentally able, may be in awe of the doctor and may not react quickly enough to ask relevant questions when they are examined or may not know what questions to ask. If you are not a relative but are the principal carer, it is important to make this clear, especially if you have Power of Attorney, as you may otherwise find that you are not given full information.

Many health authorities now have a system, variously named ('Hospital passport' and 'This is me' are two names in use) whereby the person admitted to hospital can bring with her/him a previously prepared chart which states some personal history, some likes and dislikes and some important personal information. In theory this is kept with the medical charts at the end of the bed and consulted by the nursing and care staff. This is an excellent idea but does depend on up-to-date information being provided in the first place and the care staff actually reading the document whilst attending to the patient.

Leaving hospital

The length of time the person you care for spends in hospital obviously will depend upon the injury or health problem and on how quickly s/he recovers. However, it is unlikely that s/he will be allowed home until some assessment has been made of the home circumstances. Social services will be consulted by the hospital staff if they consider your cared-for to be a 'vulnerable adult' and they may become involved at this stage even if they have not been before. An occupational therapy (OT) assessment of the home may be made to see if your cared-for can cope on discharge. If you have any doubts about her/his ability to do so, you should voice them to the OT team. If the person you care for is taken on a visit home for an assessment, try to be there as you may notice things that the OT team, however vigilant and well trained, may not.

****

My mother was desperate to leave hospital after her stroke. She was taken home for a couple of hours and the OT team assessed to see if she could get around, make a hot drink and had adequate help for getting meals and keeping the house clean. But they didn't notice that Mum could no longer manage to get in and out of bed because her leg was so weak. I don't blame them for this because Mum assured them that she could manage and even said that one of us would always be around to help her. Of course we couldn't be there all the time. Looking back, I wish we had been present at the assessment because being used to helping her around the house we might have noticed things they did not.

****

If the person you care for could manage at home with just a little extra help to begin with, then it is possible that s/he might be eligible to receive help from the reablement or intermediate care team (terminology differs in different areas), which is available through social services, through the district nursing team or through direct referral from the hospital. The aim of this help is to get people out of hospital and back home sooner than would otherwise be the case. The team will be able to supply care assistants to help with simple everyday personal care including meal preparation up to three times a day for up to 14 days. If you, or the person you care for, feel this help is appropriate and it is not offered, then make enquiries about it. Sometimes you have to pay for this care.

An alternative to going straight home is to be admitted to a local community hospital or to a care/nursing home for a convalescent period. If you feel this is necessary, you may have to be quite insistent. Unfortunately, beds in community hospitals are in high demand and a place in a care/nursing home may be available only if you are prepared to pay. However, do not be put off if you really feel that you and your cared-for will not be able to cope at home. Local authorities and social services have what is known as a 'duty of care' and they really must make a proper assessment and offer adequate help. You may find that subtle pressure is put upon you by the hospital, who will want to free up their beds as soon as possible and are impatient with 'bed-blockers'. They too have targets to meet. But your concern is with the safety and comfort of the person you care for.

****

My mother-in-law was admitted to hospital following a fall. At first she seemed to be recovering, but then her condition deteriorated and it became obvious that she would not be able to go back home. At this point the hospital began to put a lot of pressure on us to get her moved to a nursing home, but it wasn't that easy. We had to check the homes out first and make all the arrangements financially for her. On several occasions when we visited, one or other of the doctors would mention that she was taking

*up a much-needed bed, but there was no way that we could speed
things up. I realise that hospital beds are for acute cases and I feel
there should be some kind of 'halfway house' temporary arrangement in cases like ours. Of course this was a few years ago and
things may have changed now.*

****

Your cared-for's GP may be very helpful here. He or she will
have more knowledge than you of the local facilities for hospital
care and may also be able to put pressure on the hospital if you
feel that your cared-for is being discharged too soon.

****

*When my father-in-law had an accident and was taken to the local
A&E department, they wanted to discharge him back home that
evening. The trouble was that the care package he had been having had been withdrawn as soon as he was taken to hospital (he
was under the care of the intermediate care team and obviously
they were needed elsewhere), so he would have been sent home
without any care. In a bit of a panic I telephoned his doctor and he
contacted the hospital. My father-in-law was admitted to hospital
overnight until we could get everything sorted out the next day.*

****

When the person you care for is finally discharged, all the relevant
people should be informed by the hospital discharge team – for
example, the district nursing team, the carers' agency, and social
services. It is worth your contacting any vital services to be sure that
this has happened. You could also try to insist that your relative/
friend is not discharged just before a weekend because some of the
support teams will not have their full services available then.

Chapter 7

Dealing with dementia

One of the most difficult things to admit to oneself is that a loved one is becoming demented, even if all the signs are obvious to others. Dementia is also one of the most difficult things to deal with when caring for a relative, friend or neighbour.

As noted in Chapter 6, Recognising medical conditions, there are two major recognised types of dementia in the elderly, although both can be present at once. Alzheimer's disease is the one most people have heard of and it accounts for approximately 60 per cent of cases. Vascular dementia (often associated with a series of strokes) accounts for about 15 to 20 per cent. There are other, less common, forms of dementia, such as Lewy body dementia and fronto-temporal lobe dementia, and dementia can also result from a number of other, much more rare diseases and conditions. A dementia-like condition can result from certain nutritional deficiencies. If the person you care for has been diagnosed with one of the other primary causes of dementia, such as Huntington's disease, then it is likely you are already well aware of what this means.

Some medical conditions which are treatable can have symptoms similar to those of dementia, which is why a definitive diagnosis is essential if you suspect it in the person you are caring for. There are also medical treatments for dementia which can slow the progress of the disease in some people and enable them to live independent lives for longer.

Dementia is progressive and gets worse over time. Symptoms

are mild in the early stages and the carer can do a lot to help. Chapter 6 suggests signs which might indicate dementia. Although a diagnosis of dementia may make families or friends decide that the person they care for should move to a care or nursing home, this is not always the best answer in the early stages. Studies have shown that people with mild to moderate dementia go downhill less quickly when they are kept in familiar surroundings and cared for by people they know. This chapter suggests ways in which you, the carer, can help the person who has dementia and also ways in which you can make life easier for yourself and anyone else involved in their care.

Memory loss/forgetfulness

It is difficult to comprehend the 'memory loss' of dementia. It is not like the normal 'where did I put my keys?' lapses which we all suffer from occasionally. People who suffer from dementia might, for example, fail to recognize someone they know well or sometimes forget where they live, which is one reason why you often hear stories of elderly people 'wandering'.

****

We used often to see an elderly neighbour walking the streets near us and would exclaim at how active he was and how good it was that he kept fit by taking walks. Then one day he approached us when we were walking by and said, 'Excuse me, can you tell me where I live?' It appeared that he would regularly forget the way home and keep walking around until something sparked off his memory and he found his way back. It was an eye-opener for us as he had always appeared quite alert when we greeted him. We had had no idea that he was so confused.

****

Chapter 7

The memory loss associated with dementia appears to be spasmodic at first so that the person concerned might forget the way home one day but be perfectly all right the next. People with dementia may actually forget what some objects are or what their purpose is. As you would expect, items which are used most often are more likely to be remembered than those which are not.

****

I remember my sheer amazement when I first realised the extent of my mother's memory loss. I asked her for the spare car keys (she was a non-driver) and because I knew her habits suggested that she look first in her handbag. She went through each item in her handbag one by one asking me, 'Is this the car key?' even about items like business cards or her comb. It was one of the most upsetting episodes in our relationship.

****

Many people with dementia forget the day or the date. They may ask you frequently what day or date it is, or alternatively they may argue with you and flatly deny the facts. When you say that it is Saturday, for example, they may insist that it is Monday.

Some people with dementia will deny events that have clearly occurred. This is because they have no memory of them. They will perhaps claim that you haven't visited them for several days when you have actually called every day.

In the early stages much can be done to help memory lapses. But be prepared for many repetitions and the re-covering of old ground. For example, you might accompany your cared-for on a local walk and point out one or two memorable landmarks which might help her/him find the way home. 'See, there is the post office. Now we only have a few houses and then we get to your home.' Or, 'When you see that big oak tree you will know that you are nearly home.' The person you care for is quite likely to say something to the effect that, 'I know that', but it is worth persevering. The constant repetition and pointing out of landmarks might save her/him wandering many miles one day.

A useful idea is to buy a large wall calendar and encourage the person you care for to cross off the date every evening before bed, or every morning after breakfast. Then if s/he forgets the date, it can be checked on the calendar. This will only work if you are able to instil the habit of crossing off the date.

Another idea is to show the person you care for where the day and date are printed on the daily newspaper. S/he can always check the date that way, but again you will need to instil the habit of looking there. However as time progresses the date and day have less and less meaning so that even if s/he can read the date on a newspaper, for example, there is no understanding of the relevance.

You can encourage remembrance of events by gentle reminders. 'I came to see you yesterday, remember, and we ate some chocolate éclairs for tea.' Or, 'We went out together yesterday and did the shopping. Remember you bought those bananas.' Material reminders around the house will often, when pointed out, trigger the lost memory. Simple card games like Snap, and Pairs are a help to the memory too, as are games like Scrabble and noughts-and-crosses, and doing jigsaws.

Confusing time

People suffering from either form of dementia may become confused about the time of day. Strangely, this does not usually mean that they lose the ability to read the time from a clock. Indeed, if asked they may tell you the time and take a pride in being able to do so, but the actual concept of the hour of the day means nothing to them. Even the fact that it is dark or daylight may not convince them that it is night or day. You may first notice this effect particularly in the autumn as the days grow shorter and the confusion may improve in spring – but it may not.

Chapter 7

****

My mother-in-law went through a period of ringing us up in the early hours of the morning and announcing that she was just cooking dinner – or had just got dressed – or was waiting to go shopping. No amount of telling on our part would convince her that it was night or that she should go back to bed. She would say, 'I don't want to go to bed. I'm just making myself some chicken and chips,' or some other bizarre (to us) reply. Conversely, sometimes the assistant from the care agency would call at midday and Mother-in-law would refuse to answer the door because she had just gone to bed.

****

It can help here to link an event with a common occurrence rather than naming a time. For example, you could say, 'We are going shopping after such-and-such a television programme', or 'I have to go home after we have had tea'.

Telephoning or wandering the streets at night are more difficult to deal with. You can try explaining that if it is dark it is not a good idea to go out, but darkness and light have less and less significance. You can also be as short as possible when answering a night-time telephone call, but it may not have an effect. There is some research evidence that full-spectrum 'daylight' lighting used for several hours in the early part of the day can help to 'reset' the body clock and ensure a good night's sleep. You can purchase full-spectrum daylight bulbs (the light is white and really does resemble daylight) and replace the bulbs in the room which is used most during the day to see if this helps. Do not use these bulbs in the bedroom for obvious reasons.

Neglecting personal care

Over time people with dementia may begin to neglect their personal needs, such as the need to wash, to change their clothes and to eat properly. They are not being lazy as relatives often think, and a carer pointing out that they are dirty or unwashed is more likely to make them angry and resentful than to make them take the necessary action. The fact is that some people with dementia can actually forget how to do these everyday actions. They may also forget how to dress themselves and begin wearing a strange assortment of garments.

****

My father stopped bathing and shaving. At first he would wash and shave if I took him to the bathroom and insisted, but then he started resisting. I discovered that if I started the activity – put the razor into his hand and turned him towards the mirror – he would carry on. It seemed that he was just not able to initiate things – as if he didn't know how to start.

****

Some activities will be continued more than others and there does not seem to be a standard pattern. For example, the person you care for may still undress and carefully hang clothes on hangers but may not be able to find fresh clothes in the wardrobe without prompting. Or s/he may change her/his clothes but hide the soiled garments rather than putting them in the laundry basket. Some people forget to undress at all and get into bed with all their clothes on.

There are many ways you can help your relative/friend/ neighbour to cope, and in the early stages helping her/him to manage as much as possible independently will increase self-esteem as well as saving you time and trouble.

It is best not to ask people with dementia if, for example, they would like a bath or a wash. They will very likely say no. Instead, lead them to the bath after you have filled it and begin to help them remove their clothing if necessary. Or walk them to the shower, turn it on and ask them which soap they would like to use. Remember that bathing/showering every day is not absolutely necessary for cleanliness, though incontinence of course can make this more of an issue. Daily bathing or showering is a relatively modern habit and a thorough wash will do just as well. If certain parts of the body, such as between the legs, under the arms and the face and hands, are washed regularly, an all-over bath or shower can be delayed until convenient. If necessary, help to initiate the action of washing and then step back and see if the person you care for can continue alone.

Routines such as washing hair, which involve a little more effort and which are not necessarily done every day, may be neglected sooner than daily routines. The person you care for may claim that her/his hair does not need washing or perhaps even that it has already been washed. Again, it is good to remember that previous standards do not need to apply. Hair can be washed about once a fortnight provided it is thoroughly brushed/combed each day. Some people find leaning forwards over a basin uncomfortable or frightening. You could try washing hair in the shower or letting the person concerned sit in a chair and lean backwards over the basin. A large towel wrapped around her/him will mean that wet clothes do not become a problem. Some people with dementia will resist washing hair themselves but see a visit to the hairdresser as a treat, so you could arrange a regular appointment.

Washing feet and cutting toenails is another chore often forgotten or avoided, particularly if the person concerned has trouble bending forwards. It is possible to buy sponges on long sticks for use when washing the feet but those with dementia may not be able to learn how to use such aids. Suggest a weekly 'beauty treatment' which could involve washing the feet, applying foot cream and trimming the nails. If the person you are caring for can afford it, you could arrange a regular visit from a chiropodist. (Chiropodists will provide free nail care to elderly persons who have another medical condition, such as diabetes.)

When tackling problems with dressing you can try laying out clean clothes in the order in which they will be put on. Avoid complicated fastenings which may be difficult for rheumatic hands. However, many people with dementia can remember familiar actions, such as doing up buttons and zips, for a long time. Make sure that clothing is loose and comfortable and take notice if the person you are caring for shows an aversion for a particular garment. In such a case do not insist on them wearing it. You can purchase clothing which is easier to put on, such as pull-on trousers and skirts with elasticated waists, but the person concerned may prefer the type of clothing s/he is used to.

Refusal to recognise the needs of others

People with dementia are often unable to understand that others have needs as well as themselves. They may begin to appear self-ish and demanding. If you are caring for two elderly people living together and one of the partnership begins to develop dementia you may feel the need to defend the non-demented partner to the other. 'Dad isn't being unkind, Mum – he just can't manage to help you cook.' This is probably a waste of time. If possible it is best to ignore complaints and to support the non-demented partner in doing likewise. Taking the non-demented partner out regularly or arranging for the one with dementia to attend a day centre will give much-needed breaks.

If you are caring for an elderly person living alone who begins to develop dementia, s/he may start to complain that you or others are neglecting her/him even when this is untrue. Again, there is very little point in defending yourself or others. Try instead to maintain your sense of balance. Those with dementia cannot help themselves and do not understand the stress that they are causing. You in turn should not feel guilty about your own feelings of annoyance because you are doing the best you can to care for them. You may also feel guilty because you lose your temper sometimes, but do remember the sufferer will forget your cross words sooner than you do. It is very useful to 'sound off' sometimes to a friend whom you can trust. It may be best to avoid using another family member for this purpose as emotions are likely to be already very mixed in the family. You may also find the support of a local carers' group valuable. Try to give yourself regular respite time and holidays from caring if at all possible (see Chapter 8, Caring for the carer).

Fears and delusions

Irrational fears may be an early sign of dementia. For example, the person you care for may begin to keep doors locked or put furniture in front of external doors to 'stop anyone getting in', which could of course prove dangerous if emergency help is needed. S/he may begin to refuse to use one room in the house or to allow you to enter that room. S/he may claim that an innocent person like the postman is being a bother in some way. Your reassurance may help for a time but because of the memory lapses which are common with dementia, s/he may not remember your explanations for long. Insisting that s/he enters a room or leaves a door open may make her/him very nervous and cause a bad reaction. Increase the sense of security by allowing her/him to keep doors or windows closed unless it is necessary to open them. (You can open windows to air the house whilst you are present and close them when you leave, allowing the person you care for to check they are closed, perhaps). Make sure that you have keys to the house in case the person you care for refuses to answer the front door. If s/he does begin to refuse to open the door, you should make sure that any door chain is removed or you may find yourself locked out even though you have your keys. Sometimes arranging a special 'ringing code' will ensure that the person concerned answers the telephone if you call. Of course, you may have to repeat instructions for this dozens of times.

Sometimes people with dementia develop a fear that seems completely inexplicable, such as a fear of a piece of furniture or of a particular flower or scent. One important thing to remember is that eyesight is frequently affected with all forms of dementia, and particularly in dementia with Lewy bodies. The person with dementia may see shadows as people lurking, or mistake dark shapes for small animals or insects. They may find it difficult to step between different floor surfaces (such as moving from floor tiles to a carpeted area) as they perceive the surfaces to be at different heights.

****

My mother-in-law was afraid to sleep in the bed after my father-in-law died. At first she slept in the spare room, but later she avoided going to bed at all, preferring to spend the night in her reclining armchair. It took a while before we realised this was happening; only piecing together snippets of conversation and 'clues' from the cleaning lady made us realise. It became clear that she had had 'an accident' and wet the bed once. This was not a regular occurrence but it had frightened her enough to put her off using the bed. I brought a mattress cover and spent a long time showing it to her and explaining that this would protect the mattress if anything of the sort happened again. Eventually she did sleep in the bed again, but she occasionally reverted to sleeping in the chair if anything had upset her.

****

The simplest thing to do, if reassurance doesn't work, is to allow the fear without agreeing with it. In other words, avoid buying that particular flower or using that scent, and move the piece of furniture out of the way. There is no need to agree that the fear is rational but trying to convince someone that their fears are unreal seldom works and is likely only to cause anger and resentment.

People with dementia may appear to have delusions, but it is often difficult to tell if these are real delusions or are just the result of 'confabulation'. The person you care for may say that s/he has received a visit from someone when you know this to be untrue. It may be that s/he is under the delusion that someone has visited but it may just be that s/he has come upon a cup of tea which s/he had forgotten about and has filled in the memory lapse by confabulating a story about someone coming to tea. Or it may be that a memory from the past has surfaced and s/he is simply describing what happened then. Sometimes the stories are very strange and often they concern long-lost relatives visiting. People with dementia seem to lose later memories before earlier ones and so may insist that a deceased son, daughter or husband is still alive and even that they are frequent callers. There does appear to be a tendency for the brain in those with short-term memory loss to 'fill in the gaps' when recalling something and this may account for some 'delusions'.

However, some forms of dementia (especially Lewy body dementia) may cause more frequent visual effects and sometimes these take the form of hallucinations. These are very real to the person who sees them and it is usually NOT helpful to try to 'reason' them away by taking the person experiencing the hallucinations and showing her/him, say, an empty chair and saying, for example, 'Look, there is no one there'. The person experiencing the hallucinations is likely to just be very upset and refuse to believe you. In these circumstances it is best to 'go along' with the idea. You do not have to agree that the visual effects are real. It is easy to say when told that someone is sitting on the sofa something like, 'Oh well, let's leave them there and go into the kitchen for our tea'. Such an action is less stressful for you, the carer, and it is certainly less stressful for the person experiencing the hallucination.

Difficulty with conversation and loss of speech

This manifests itself in a variety of different ways depending on the individual. One major difficulty seems to be an inability to tell you something in a way that makes sense, even though the ability to talk is unimpaired. For example, the person you care for may try to explain that someone has telephoned: 'The bell rang…Sally…very loud…coming today…yesterday.' Or s/he may substitute a word which has associations with what they are trying to say: 'We went out to the grass' (meaning, garden). This type of difficulty calls for a lot of patience from the carer. You may have to spend a lot of time trying to unravel the meaning from a jumble of phrases, especially if the person you care for is upset about something and you feel that you really need to get to the bottom of what it is. Over time you may learn to understand the 'word associations' your relative or friend uses, but this may not remain consistent since dementia is progressive.

One idea is to try to get your relative or friend to lead you to where s/he wants to go or to point to what s/he means. For example, s/he might point to the telephone if relaying news of a telephone call. It might help you to write down key words as you 'unravel' what the story is so that you keep to the point and don't get led astray by irrelevancies. In the example above about the telephone, the phrase 'very loud' is not significant but 'coming today' probably is. It may take several attempts for you to understand and the person concerned may just give up the effort if you press too hard.

You could also try to relax her/him and pick up the thread again later by referring to the matter in a gentle tone. Anxiety tends to confuse people with dementia and they are likely to be put off if you convey your own worry to them or if you try to press or 'browbeat' them into explanations. Remember too that certain concepts may be conveyed correctly even though the words are wrong. The person concerned might say 'park' instead of garden or 'taxi' instead of 'bus', but the inherent meaning is there.

****

My mother said one day, 'My cousin came to see me yesterday – my girl cousin.' Well, to our knowledge Mum had no cousin left alive, but after I thought about it a little I asked her, 'Do you mean that your sister came to see you? Jeannie?' She was delighted that I had understood. She knew it was a relative but the only word for a relation she could recall at that moment was cousin.

****

Another major difficulty may be in the understanding of speech. The person you care for may not respond at all when you ask a question. This is because s/he is unable to make sense of what you are asking.

A frequent problem is when people with dementia respond 'No' to every question. They may not understand what is being asked, but somehow they seem to sense that a question often involves something they don't want to make the effort to do. Or they may sense that replying 'No' often makes the questioner give up and stop bothering them. Occasionally a person with dementia answers 'Yes' to every question instead, or 'Yes' and 'No' at random. The best way around this is not to ask questions unless really necessary. Instead of 'Would you like to go into the garden?' say, 'Let's go into the garden now', perhaps taking their arm and leading them, gently. Instead of 'Would you like a cup of tea?' say, 'I'll make you a cup of tea now'.

When you have to explain something use short sentences and simple language: 'We are going for a walk now', not, 'I thought we'd go out for a walk after you've eaten your lunch. It's really quite cold so you'll need your coat, but I can fetch it later'.

It is also worth reinforcing your words with actions – fetching the walking stick if you are suggesting a walk or offering the plate of cake when asking if s/he would like a cake. It also helps to use body language: 'Is your foot hurting?' (touching the foot and looking concerned).

Sometimes people with dementia retain a social veneer which enables them to maintain a conversation, but if you carry the conversation beyond the simple 'social' level they are unable to respond. However, the social veneer is very valuable and can be helpful to the self-respect of the person with dementia.

****

When I first employed a professional carer to help look after my sister I had trouble convincing her on the first visit that there was anything wrong. My sister made the tea and sat talking with us, even making voluntary remarks about the weather or a TV programme she liked to watch. It was only as the carer began to visit regularly that she realised that my sister would use the same phrases on every occasion. It was always 'a lovely day', or she 'loved the gardening programme'.

Even when having a conversation is difficult, the effort of doing so can be helpful to your relative or friend. Talking about familiar things and naming common objects helps to retain speech and understanding as long as possible. You could, for example, name things as you go along in as natural a way as possible: 'We'll put the sandwiches on this plate and the cake on this plate. If you carry the sandwiches in, I will bring the cake.'

Looking at photographs and watching video tapes of past events is very helpful, both as an aid to memory and as an aid to speech: 'Oh look, there's Andy kicking the ball. He looks happy.' 'Do you remember when that rose bush was against the wall there? It was a lovely colour.'

Another element of not understanding speech is the loss of the ability to understand the written word. Surprisingly, many people with dementia can still read perfectly well; they just cannot understand what they are reading.

****

When my mother was in hospital they used to bring round the menu cards for her to choose her meals. She would proudly read out to me: 'Breakfast: choose two; orange juice, porridge, toast...', but she was quite unable to choose what she wanted unless I translated by asking her in simple terms, 'Would you like toast for breakfast?' Often someone with dementia might seem to be reading a magazine you have provided, but if you talk about any of the articles it becomes clear that they do not understand what they have read.

****

Incontinence

Incontinence is discussed in Chapter 6, Recognising medical conditions. When people suffer from dementia they often become incontinent and it is often listed by carers as one of the most difficult things to deal with. At first a person with mild dementia seems to understand and to be upset and embarrassed by incontinence, and at this stage you will probably find that s/he tries to hide 'accidents'. Later s/he may appear to ignore or even to be unaware of it. When someone is only mildly demented it may be possible to explain to them the use of incontinence pads and pants and what to do with their wet or soiled clothes, but you should still be ready for odd lapses of memory.

****

I began to notice a smell of urine on my visits to my mother. She denied any problem and always said that she couldn't smell anything herself. She didn't like me poking around the house so it wasn't until one day when my brother had taken her out shopping that I got the chance to have a good look around. I found dozens of items of underwear, towels and old rags stuffed behind the radiators. She had obviously cleaned up after her 'accidents' and then tried to hide the 'evidence'. Luckily she was still able to understand how to cope after I had explained to her what to do and provided her with proper incontinence clothing. I did find that she had the odd lapse, but the smell would alert me and I would simply go through the instructions with her again. She was able to just about cope until her death.

****

It is a waste of time, as well as unkind, to get annoyed when someone with dementia suffers from incontinence. They really cannot help their 'accidents'. However, it is worth having them checked over by the doctor because urinary infections can sometimes cause temporary incontinence, which will resolve when the infection clears up. It is also worth investing in clothes with simple fastenings which are washable. Sometimes incontinence is simply the result of not getting to the lavatory in time. In cases like this, taking the person concerned to the toilet regularly may help to avoid accidents.

Frequently the onset of incontinence is the 'last straw' that causes families, or friends, to contemplate helping the person they care for to move to a nursing home. It can be some consolation in these circumstances to remind yourself that the person you care for will at least be kept clean, dry and comfortable as nursing home staff are used to dealing with the problem and have the facilities and equipment to cope.

The Mental Health Act

You often hear talk of 'locking someone up' or hear someone thoughtlessly say, 'He ought to be put away for his own protection'. However, dementia alone is not a legal reason to restrict someone's liberty.

The Mental Capacity Act came fully into force on 1 October 2007. It aims to protect people who cannot make decisions for themselves due to a learning disability or a mental health condition, or for any other reason. A lack of capacity could be because of dementia. The Act provides clear guidelines for carers and professionals about who can take decisions in which situations. The Act states that everyone should be treated as able to make their own decisions until it is shown that they cannot. It also aims to enable people to make their own decisions for as long as they are capable of doing so. A person's capacity to make a decision will be established at the time that a decision needs to be made. So someone might, for example, have capacity to decide whether s/he wishes to go on an outing but not have the capacity to decide about moving into a care home. The Act also provides protection to anyone lacking capacity as it makes it a criminal offence to neglect or ill-treat a person who lacks capacity.

The social services department of each local authority has a duty of care for vulnerable adults living in its area. It has to assess the needs of these adults and provide services and/or equipment to meet any assessed needs. This means that if the social care workers believe that a person's care needs can no longer be met at home, they may be able to place that person in an environment where her/his care needs can be met, such as a care home.

If the social workers and any doctors involved consider that someone with dementia can no longer be cared for at home, they will first try to persuade her/him to go into a care home voluntarily. However, some people with dementia don't believe that they have a problem and are reluctant to leave their home. Striking a balance between their safety and freedom and the safety of others is not easy.

The principles of the Mental Capacity Act include supporting people to make decisions for themselves wherever possible, and making decisions in the best interests of people who don't have mental capacity (see above). The Code of Practice which accompanies the Act outlines how health professionals should support the person and/or include carers in the decision-making process.

Admission to hospital, under mental health legislation, might only need to be on a temporary basis, while measures are taken to circumvent such problems – for example, automatic electrical switches can be fitted which switch off cookers, irons, etc after a limited time period, and regular assistance can be provided to help the individual to bathe, shower, keep clean and eat. This would mean that a person with dementia might be able to return home to live after these matters have been attended to.

Chapter 8

Caring for the carer

Being a carer is very stressful and very tiring. It can also be very fulfilling and many of us are glad to be 'giving something back', especially if it is to a parent who once cared for us. But there is no denying that it can sometimes feel as though we are labouring under an intolerable burden. It is very seldom, even in the best-regulated and closest of families, that the burden of caring seems to be shared equally amongst the family members. There may be many reasons for this. Some members of the family may live too far away to give 'hands-on' care. Some may have a closer relationship than others with the person being cared for. Some people work longer hours or in more stressful jobs than others. Sometimes, sadly, certain family members do not want to be involved in the care of their relatives. Frequently, the burden of care falls on the family member, or friend if family are not involved, who lives nearest, or who is perceived as having the most time to give. It is a fact that carers are more often female than male and perhaps society sees caring as a female pursuit rather than a male one.

In general it is true to say that the role of 'carer' is not planned for or logically decided upon. In an ideal world, as our relatives or close friends grow steadily more frail, plans would be made for the future, money saved for contingencies, moves made to more manageable accommodation, and help enlisted in advance.

In the real world, people fall ill suddenly, accidents happen, sudden death happens, events overtake us and the role of carer is suddenly ours without planning or forethought. Very often there is a dramatic change in situation after the death of one member of an elderly partnership. There is a sudden realisation that the remaining partner will not be able to cope alone without substantial input from other members of the family, or friends, 'the carers'. In such an emergency, contingency plans have to be made and actions taken without there being enough time to consider the consequences.

If at all possible, time should be made after the initial 'emergency' to take a step back, draw breath and consider a 'care plan'. It is very worthwhile at this stage to get together and agree co-operation with everyone involved. Lack of this co-operation may turn out to be the biggest underlying problem. Resentment and hostility quickly build up in the absence of communication. Guilt plays a part. A daughter living some distance away may really resent the hands-on care given by a daughter-in-law even whilst knowing and understanding that she is unable to give it herself. A son may not feel at all able to give this kind of care and react by belittling the care given by his sisters.

****

We are a big family and after Dad died it is true to say that each of us took a part in looking after Mum and helping her move house and settle into her new way of life. Looking back we are all able to see that. At the time though, I don't think there was one of us who didn't at some time think that we were the one being put upon and that everyone else was 'slacking'. Some of us were more involved with the practical side of packing up the household and cleaning, others helped sort out the finances and my sister who lived furthest away and couldn't do any day-to-day business took Mum away to stay with her for the weekend on several occasions. It's only looking back that we can all see the part each of us played. At the time, shock and guilt really did interfere with clear thinking. If we hadn't been such a close family I believe we could have fallen out permanently then.

****

Group meetings early on, where concrete plans are made and (if possible) where recriminations are withheld, will help avoid such situations developing. If someone lives too far away to help with daily care, perhaps s/he can agree to come and stay at intervals and give 'holiday cover' to the chief carer. Someone who is not good at practical personal care may instead be able to manage the financial affairs. It helps to make use of personal strengths here. Someone who enjoys cooking may agree to keep the freezer stocked with ready meals whilst someone who is only free once a week but is a car driver might organise the shopping. A family member who works within the health service may act as the co-ordinator for healthcare.

There is no reason why, once the initial emergency is over, the family and friends should not hold their own regular assessments of what needs to be done and draw up their own 'care plan' at intervals. If possible, do not let the plethora of tasks which need to be done build up in a piecemeal fashion. Care needs are likely to be constantly changing. Gradually you may find that the level of care needs to be increased or changed to suit a changing state of health or disability in your relative or friend. Sometimes care needs may decrease – for example, following recuperation after a hospital admission.

****

There were five of us involved in caring for Mum and at first we were all so busy that we never found time to meet and discuss what each of us was doing. Sometimes we found we had 'doubled up' on things and other things slipped through the net because we weren't communicating. One Christmas after a family get-together we made a decision to meet up again in three months to discuss how things were going and whether we needed to make other changes. This quarterly get-together became a family reunion and we kept it up even after Mum died. We still start the day with a toast to Mum because without her we might have all drifted apart more.

****

What if you are the only family member? You should not try to take on everything alone. There may well be neighbours or friends of your relative who will help in the same way that family do. Otherwise you will have to turn to professional help. There is no need to feel guilt over this. Indeed, some elderly people prefer the notion that any help they are receiving is 'paid' help and not done as a favour. Remember that you do not have to go through social services to get professional help, although you may wish to do so (see Chapter 9 on Care agencies and professional carers).

Caring for a member of the family is an unpaid 'occupation' but you or the person you care for may be able to claim certain grants and allowances (see Chapter 2 on Financial Matters, page 29 – Benefits) and if you are entitled to them you should certainly claim them. Do not allow the person you care for, or yourself, to be put off by thoughts of 'living off the state' or claiming 'charity'. Most of us have paid into the state through National Insurance contributions and all of us are entitled to claim help from the state when we need it. There is an additional factor. Being in receipt of certain benefits often qualifies you for other financial help or gives you priority when seeking other non-cash benefits. Some benefits are means tested and the entitlement may in itself mean very little. You may think that the receipt of, say, 40p per week is not worth the effort of claiming, but the extra benefits may make it very worthwhile. An example of this is Disability Living Allowance. If the person you care for is in receipt of this allowance at the higher rate, s/he automatically qualifies for a 'Blue Badge', which allows parking in 'disabled' car park spaces. Similarly, being in receipt of Attendance allowance may entitle someone to help with council tax payments.

Conversely, receipt of certain benefits may make you or the person you care for ineligible for other benefits which might be more useful to you both, or make you financially better off. The whole benefits area is a bit of a minefield and it can be helpful to take advice from one of the organisations that specialise in giving information in this area. There are some websites which enable you to check out your eligibility (see Further useful information, page 209) or you can contact the Department of Work and Pensions benefits helpline or talk to an advisor at the Citizens' Advice Bureau.

You may not realise that, if you are a carer, you can ask the local authority for an assessment of your own needs. If you live in England or Wales you are entitled to an assessment whether or not the person you are caring for is having an assessment themselves. In Scotland you can receive an assessment only if the person you are caring for is being assessed. Except in Scotland, where there is no standard list of what should be assessed, the assessment is supposed to take into account your work, or desire to work, and your need for training, education and leisure activities. The kind of help and support you can get as a carer includes: respite care to give you a break if you are caring constantly for your relative; emotional support from other carers, usually through a local support group; help with caring; and help with household tasks and activities for the person you care for. You should also be told about any benefits you are entitled to claim. Your assessment may be made by a social worker from the local authority social services department or it may be carried out by a worker from a private agency employed on behalf of social services. It may be made over the telephone.

Before you have an assessment you might want to think about the following because these are things that you may be asked about and will perhaps need to write notes on:

- If you need to get up in the night to care for your relative or friend, are you getting enough sleep?
- Are you able to get out and do things by yourself or does the person you care for need to have someone with her/him constantly?
- Do you feel that your health is being affected by caring? For example, are you having to do any heavy lifting (physical health) or is the situation making you depressed (mental health)?
- Are you able to cope with other family commitments? Are you also having to run a home and care for husband/wife and children?
- Are you finding juggling work and caring difficult? You may have to work to earn a living and are having to fit caring in around your working day.

Talk to the person doing your assessment about these and any other issues that you think may affect your ability to continue caring. Remember that by caring for your relative or friend you are helping to maintain the current state policy of ensuring 'care in the community' and are saving the state money in terms of possible care home fees.

If you feel that you need an urgent assessment (if you suddenly have to go into hospital, for example) then make this clear to the social services Duty Officer because they are able to organise 'emergency assessments'.

In a perfect world we would receive all the help needed to care for our relative or friend through official channels and all the facilities would be there to assist us. In actual fact the level of help available varies widely from area to area. Local authorities have limited resources and have to give the help they can to those most in need based on their own assessment of where the need is greatest. So it is fairly certain that you will have to find ways and means to relieve some of the burden of caring for yourself.

First, do not neglect to ask for help from the person you care for's friends and neighbours if you need it. Carers are a huge 'silent force' within the community and many struggle on, feeling that to ask for help is a confession of weakness and inability to cope. As well as using the services of the local authority, actively seek for other informal help. Friends and neighbours may well be able and willing to fill 'gaps' in the help supplied officially. Many people are pleased and even flattered to be asked to help, but the most important advice here is to be specific. A neighbour will often promise to 'keep an eye on things' but it would be much more useful if you asked them to do something specific – say, 'Can you call round each morning just to check all is well?' or 'Could you pick up and change the library books on Thursdays?' Of course, people may sometimes be unable to help, but unless and until you ask you will never know.

****

One of the ladies at our local church suffered from vascular dementia. Her husband was quite dedicated and refused to allow her to go into a nursing home, continuing to look after her himself until just a few weeks before she died. A group of parishioners from the Senior Citizens Group got together and formed a rota to sit with the poor lady once a week so that her husband could have a few hours to himself. Sometimes he went visiting or had an outing and sometimes he just caught up on some sleep. He had some respite and she had the company of people she knew. He told me afterwards that he would not have

been able to cope without this respite and because it was done
on a rota basis no one person felt they had to take on too much.

****

Also investigate local clubs and organisations to which the person you care for belongs. If s/he belongs to a church or equivalent you will almost certainly be able to get help to transport her/him to services and perhaps a lift to any church-related clubs s/he belongs to, or you might get respite in the form of visitors or help with shopping and other errands. If s/he belongs to a local branch of an organisation such as, for example, The British Legion, ask if members can offer any help. Ex-servicemen and -women's organisations can be particularly helpful, and many elderly people are ex-service due to war service and National Service in the years that followed the Second World War. Another alternative source of help can be local branches of organisations set up to benefit ex-members of professions or trades. Some examples are given in Further useful information for this chapter (see page 216), but if you can't find the appropriate organisation there, keep investigating. Use the local library or the internet as a starting point.

Local and national charities can also be sources of help. You may think that your needs or those of the person you care for are too insignificant to be of interest to these charities, but you may be surprised to learn that some charities, far from having their resources stretched too thinly, are desperate to find those who need their help.

****

My friend was temporary Chief Executive of a charity which
gave help to those who could not afford to pay their water charg-
es. He surprised me by telling me one day that the charity had
great trouble finding people who they could help, not because

the help was not needed but because their advertising was poor and that therefore those who needed their help were not being informed that it was available for the asking.

****

As a carer, it is very important that you look after your own physical and mental health. You should take care of yourself physically by eating properly and taking exercise, but you should also build in some sensible respite (see below). If you feel you need it, make sure you also access support for yourself. There are several organisations aimed at supporting carers (see Further useful information, page 216). Some of these offer information, some offer practical support and some offer 'moral support' in the form of local support groups where carers can meet to talk about their problems or concerns with people who are in a similar situation to them. There are often separate groups which give support to carers of those suffering from dementia. Your local GP surgery will almost certainly have information about local support groups, or you can ask the district nursing team about them. Information about national carers' organisations can be obtained via the internet or from your local library. Many support organisations have carers' support chatrooms and forums accessed via their website and you may find this kind of 'virtual' support most helpful as it can be accessed out of normal working hours when you may actually have more leisure available.

It can be difficult, but try not to allow yourself to feel constantly guilty. Those who we care for do not always show their appreciation, and indeed in some cases, they may be unable to do so. Parents have grown used to nagging their children, old friends have grown used to taking help given for granted. Other members of the family may find it easier to find fault with the care you are giving rather than offering support. Try always to assure yourself that you are doing the best you can. Do not feel guilty if you sometimes feel annoyed with or speak crossly to those you care for. If you feel that your feelings may get the better of you and lead to any form of action stronger than cross words, make every attempt to stand back from the situation and seek help.

It is most important that carers consider their own health and sanity as well as that of the people they care for. You should never neglect your own health issues because if you are ill the person you are caring for will suffer as well since you will be unable to give the level of care you would wish to.

****

A friend of mine, in his 80s himself, was looking after his wife with Alzheimer's disease and refused to leave her for any length of time. He got so exhausted that he slipped down the stairs and knocked himself out, with loss of memory afterwards. After such a head injury he should have been observed in hospital for signs of bleeding inside his skull but, because of his sense of duty, he refused to be admitted. Three weeks later he had a fit and was admitted with a large blood clot on the brain and continuing bleeding. He later died and his wife had to be admitted to a residential home – the very thing he had, mistakenly, been trying to avoid.

****

If you visit your doctor for a health problem which needs a referral to an outpatient clinic or involves being referred for an operation, make sure that the doctor knows you are a carer. When referring patients, doctors take into account not only the severity of the health problem referred, but also any circumstances in the patient's life that might mean s/he should be seen more quickly than normal. This is standard practice, but your doctor cannot take the fact that you are a carer into account if he does not know that you are. These days most doctors do not know their patients personally and, although they should ask you about problems of everyday living which might be affecting your health, many do not have time to do so. So tell the doctor that you are a carer for your relative or friend, and if you are going to have to make special arrangements for their care in order to get treatment for your own health make sure that the doctor knows this. You can ask the receptionist at the surgery for a form to register the fact that you are a carer. This should then be kept with your medical notes.

If you are a full-time carer you should do your very best to build in some respite time. You might pay for a professional carer to come in and sit with your cared-for once or twice a week, or you might be able to find a friend, neighbour or other family member who will do this. You may find a local charity or other organisation who will provide this service. If you are regularly woken at night in order to care for your relative or friend, then for your own safety you should try to organise at least one night of unbroken sleep each week. There are agencies which provide a 'night sitting' service, or you could ask another member of the family to give you relief from night duty on a regular basis.

Even if you are not caring for your relative or friend full time you will want to go away on holiday occasionally. Another member of the family, or a friend or neighbour, may be prepared to take over your visiting and caring duties for the length of the holiday. The fact is that families can sometimes be quite selfish over this and so you may have to be prepared to be insistent. An alternative option is to try to arrange respite care for your relative or friend in a local care or nursing home. There can be certain difficulties over this. Although theoretically most homes offer this facility, your chosen home may not have room at the time you need it. The other possibility is that the person you care for may be quite stubborn about going away for respite care. S/he may be worried that it is 'the thin end of the wedge' and is leading up to a permanent placement in a care home, which s/he may dread. They may just not want to leave their familiar surroundings. Familiarity is an important element of independence for the elderly, particularly for those with any form of disability such as poor sight or difficulty in getting about around the house. If this is the case, try to enlist the help of other family members to persuade the person concerned that you need the break (see Chapter 10 on Managing change). Don't forget that the local authority social services department has a 'duty of care' for carers as well as for those cared for, so if you can't make informal arrangements or can't find a local care/nursing home to help, contact the Duty Officer in the social services department.

Make use of all the resources you can to help you and the person you care for. Read books, check magazine articles, ask at the library, search the internet. Buy or arrange provision of any equipment that will make life easier. Above all, ask what is available. Especially ask your district nursing team. They have access to a lot of information and contacts.

****

I was nagging my teenage son one day about some task that he hadn't done and he responded wittily with, 'Careful Dad, I'll be the one choosing your nursing home when the time comes!' It was meant as a joke of course (I think!), but it did make me start to take stock of what future I wanted for myself.

****

At this point it occurs to many carers to think about their own future. Many of us have plans for our retirement, but for most of us, in our imagination and planning this means 'active retirement'. It is very difficult to think about planning for a frail old age because most of us do not want to imagine this future. However, if you don't want to be in the position of having others make decisions for you, then make your plans now for this possible future. It is a very good time to make plans whilst you are caring for another because the difficulties and limitations of frail old age will be clearly before you (as well, perhaps, as the compensations). So, this could be an ideal time to think about the following:

- Where would you like to live and what would be the most practical accommodation? Many people have a vision of old age in a bungalow, which is why bungalows are so highly sought after. However, with modern facilities such as lifts, a small flat might be the answer. Many 'retirement' complexes are being designed and built now to cater for the ageing population and if you have the chance you could look around some and decide what is likely to suit you when the time comes.

****

We were so lucky in finding Mum a house in a 'mixed' complex. There were several small privately owned cottages, each designed for one or two elderly people, and a small block of rented flats all owned by the same Trust. There was a resident warden and a social centre and the communal gardens were all beautifully maintained. She retained her sense of independence because the house was hers but she was able to use the social facilities and had company nearby when she wanted it. However, we had quite a search to find just the right place for her and she had to go on the waiting list for several months before one of the houses came up for sale.

****

- Do you have small physical problems now (arthritis, for example) which might develop in the future and mean that you would need special aids and equipment to manage to be independent? Now is the time to look at catalogues and keep an eye on new developments in the equipment field. Now is the time to put aside money if you think expensive items of aid equipment might be needed.

- Plan for your pension. Most of us realise that the state pension is not going to be enough to live on. Personal pension planning needs to begin many years before we need it. Think ahead about nursing home fees in case they might be required. There are special plans available which mean that you can make allowances for nursing home fees whilst still maintaining as much of your capital as possible. (See Further useful information on page 217 and Chapter 2 on Financial matters.)

- Make a will. Many people believe that if they do not make a Will their next of kin will automatically get all their estate. This does not happen. See Chapter 12 on Wills and probate.

- Think about arranging Power of Attorney in case you need it. It doesn't have to be implemented until you want to but it has to be drawn up whilst you are able to understand what you are doing and can sign the documents. Do not be put off. This does not only mean thinking in terms of dementia but considering what would be the needs of your family if, for example, you suffered a stroke and could not sign cheques or use your debit card.

- Why not spend time getting to know about the kinds of care homes and nursing homes available and even look at one or two just in case. If in the future you need this level of care, why let others decide for you then when you can make your own decisions now.

- Write down your wishes for the future. Discuss them with your next of kin, your family and your friends. Don't let people tell you that you are being morbid. Explain that it will make their lives easier if they know what you want to happen if you get very frail.

- Don't get depressed by all this forward thinking. Feel secure in that you have made all the plans you possibly can.

Chapter 9

Care agencies and professional carers

Mum could manage the routine housework even though she couldn't see very well, but we needed to get some regular help for 'difficult' jobs, such as cleaning the windows, vacuuming under the bed, and trimming the hedges in the garden. She could afford to pay and I thought it would be a simple matter to find a handy person who would come in regularly. But I was amazed to find how particular the agencies were. Some would do only 'light housework' and some would do internal chores but nothing in the garden. In the end we had to have a mix of options and my sister and I took over the difficult vacuuming by taking it in turns once each week.

****

Sooner or later you or the person for whom you are caring may begin to consider the need for professional carers to help on a regular basis. It may be that you live too far away to carry out your caring duties on a daily basis. Or perhaps you have a job which prevents you being able to carry out much physical daily care. It may be that the needs of the person you care for have developed beyond what you and other family members or friends are able to provide.

In theory, local authority social services departments are

responsible for arranging services to help older and disabled people stay in their own homes. Many people believe that they have to get this sort of help through social services or that social services will recommend a care agency. In fact, you are perfectly at liberty to make your own private arrangements and you can contact a care agency direct without involving social services. Although the local authority social services department may furnish you with a list of approved or inspected agencies, they will not usually make a specific recommendation.

Getting help through social services

If you or the person you care for decide to arrange help via social services, this is the procedure. The first step towards arranging home-care services is for you or the person you care for to contact your local council social services department for an **'assessment of needs'** to be undertaken. This assessment is sometimes known as a **'community care assessment'**. The social services department is supposed to react in a timely manner according to the urgency involved. If, for example, you have suddenly fallen ill and your relative needs immediate help, then the Duty Officer in the local department ought to be able to call on someone to provide help immediately. On the other hand, if you are just making enquiries about what help might be needed at a future date, your need will be assessed as much less urgent. Be aware, however, that each department reacts differently according to its efficiency and the calls that it already has on its resources, as well as on its assessment of the urgency of the case. If you do not feel that you are getting a service that is fast enough, be prepared to keep calling and keep insisting that your need is urgent.

The assessment process will examine the needs of the person you care for and how these can be met. During an assessment, the person you care for (and you, if you choose to be present, and you should arrange this if you possibly can) will be asked questions about her/his circumstances, the situations and activities s/he finds difficult, and any support being received from family, friends, neighbours and the local community.

The assessment process should involve other professionals, such as the GP or the district nurse, or anyone who has been closely connected with providing care. The social worker doing the assessment should provide you with information about what support is available locally, so that you can make a choice about how the needs of the person you care for should be met. This information may be as simple as telling you to call in a local cleaning agency (which social services may employ on your behalf), or suggesting you check your local Yellow Pages for a window cleaner. On the other hand, it may point you to useful local services that can provide for any useful specific needs.

At the end of the assessment process you and/or the person you care for should be provided with a clearly written statement declaring what the needs are, how these needs will be met and which organisations or individuals can be involved in meeting those needs, together with their contact details. This statement is called the 'care plan'.

At this point there can also be an assessment of your cared-for's finances, which will look at both income and capital savings to see how much s/he can afford to pay towards services provided by the local council. There are wide variations in how much is charged. However, government guidance states that charges must be 'reasonable' and must not cause undue financial hardship.

You can get further details about charges from various websites or telephone helplines (see Chapter 2 which includes Entitlements, benefits and how to apply for them – see page 19). If the person you care for is not financially able to make any contribution to the cost of care services but is clearly in need of them, the local authority may fund these. However, there is virtually no direct provision these days of what used to be known as 'home help'. In cases where the local authority will fund help they will contract with a private agency to provide the care and pay the agency direct. 'Home helps' directly employed by the local authority are a thing of the past.

However, councils also have a duty to offer the choice of direct payments to all individuals who have been assessed as needing services and who meet certain criteria. The **Direct Payments Scheme** means that the person you care for can directly receive funds to 'employ' her/his own support, rather than having services directly supplied by the council.

Generally speaking, if the person you care for can afford to do so, s/he will have to pay something towards professional caring services whether you arrange these via social services or privately. Agency fees are usually quoted on an hourly basis and include administration charges. The general rule seems to be that the actual care worker receives between one third and one half of the fee you pay to the agency.

Arranging professional carers privately

It is neither as quick nor as simple to call in a professional caring agency as you might think. Therefore it is a good idea to begin your research as soon as you start to think such services might be needed, even if it appears that that date is some time in the future.

This chapter gives some general advice about where to start when researching professional care, and some information that will help to save time and trouble during the actual process of arranging care. There are various different types of agency and before contacting any it is good to make a list of what specific help is likely to be needed. This helps you to narrow down the list of agency contacts and to give specific information to the agency when you do make the contact.

Broadly, professional caring falls into four main areas: nursing care, cleaning and household duties, companionship and personal care.

Nursing care

It is possible to obtain private nursing care in your own home and there are agencies who specialise in hiring out nurses for this purpose. Such care is usually very expensive and if your relative is sick enough to require nursing care at home it is very possible that it is available through the National Health Service (NHS), so make careful investigations first, unless you specifically want to use private care. Your local NHS provider can supply help with:

- incontinence advice and equipment
- chiropody
- occupational therapy
- physiotherapy
- medical equipment, such as wheelchairs and special beds.

Care for patients with a specific illness, such as cancer or multiple sclerosis, can also sometimes be available through the NHS. To find out what is available in your area approach your relative/friend's GP, or the District Nursing Service.

Professional agency nurses are usually very specific about the services that they will and will not provide and the agencies through which you obtain this care will explain this to you. In general, do not expect a professional nurse to deal with personal care, such as bathing or helping with dressing, or with any form of housework or cooking.

Cleaning and household duties

There are agencies that will provide people to tackle cleaning and housework, but if this is the only sort of help your relative/friend needs, you may prefer to make a private arrangement with an individual cleaner. Agency fees tend to be very high for this type of work. However, hiring through an agency will ensure that you get continuous cover during holiday times or sickness, and the agency will take care of PAYE and National Insurance matters for you. They will also follow up the references of their workers and in many cases do a Disclosure and Barring Service (DBS) check; you may feel that it is worth paying for this convenience. A cleaning agency will usually do an initial survey of your needs and will provide a written document stating what services will be provided. You may be surprised to discover that private cleaning services, whether through an individual or an agency, can be quite particular about what they will and will not do. Some cleaning services will not make beds or change bed linen, for example. Many cleaners refuse to do 'heavy work', such as cleaning windows. The unfortunate thing is that frail elderly people can often cope with routine daily chores and it is with the 'heavy work' that they need the help.

****

My parents already had a cleaner whom they trusted and who seemed willing and competent. So when it became a problem for Mum to change the duvet cover I thought it would be simple to ask the cleaner to extend her duties to include this. I was amazed when she told me that she 'did not do beds'.

****

Companionship

You can actually pay for 'companionship' – that is, having a more able-bodied person around most of the time or for specific periods – and some agencies specialise in this type of service. You might choose this option if the person you care for is housebound or has an otherwise restricted social life, and if you and the rest of the family or other friends are unable to supply all that is needed to combat loneliness or other social needs. These paid companions will usually do light shopping and collect prescriptions or library books. They will also take the person you care for on outings or stay at home with her/him and keep her/him company, playing card games, chatting and being available, say, to answer the door when tradesmen call. Some agencies will provide carers who give a companionship service in combination with cleaning or personal care. Again, you will need to make careful enquiries.

Personal care

Carers from agencies who provide this service will help with things like getting in and out of bed, bathing and washing, and dressing, as well as preparing meals, shopping and cleaning. Depending upon your needs, some agencies will also provide staff to give medicines, stoke solid-fuel stoves, defrost freezers and turn their hand to whatever needs doing.

Choosing an agency

Once you have narrowed down exactly which services you require you can begin researching care agencies. There are a number of options when it comes to finding the right one.

- You may be able to get details of approved private agencies from your local social services department. Ask for the Company Registration department. Remember that they are not usually allowed to recommend a specific agency.
- You may get a recommendation from a friend or relative. This can be very helpful as you will be able to get an idea of the standard of care received and also of the quality of administrative handling (see below).
- You can use the internet or the local telephone directory and find care agencies in your area. At first there will seem to be a bewildering number available to help you with care. In fact you may find that your choices are much more limited. The web pages or telephone book may have a long list of names but often all four types of caring agency are lumped together under a generic term such as 'Nursing and Care Agencies', meaning that you will first have to sift the list to extract only those that provide

the services you require. To increase the difficulty, many agencies do not specify in their advertisements what type of care they provide. You may have to make several initial investigatory calls just to narrow your search to those who will provide what you require.

- The UK Home Care Association (contact details on page 217) can give you details of home care providers who follow their code of practice.

Practicalities

Find an agency that works in your area: Many advertise that they give a countrywide service (they are part of a chain or operate franchises); others operate only locally. Here again you may have to speak to them to pin down availability. The initial advertisement might indicate that the agency supplies services throughout your county but when enquiring you may find that they cannot supply your particular area because they do not have carers either living, or willing to travel, there. Of course, there is more likely to be a problem in rural areas and especially if you need carers to come to an isolated village or house.

Plan the times and days you need help: You need to consider whether the person you care for needs help every day (with washing and dressing, for example) or only once or twice a week (for cleaning and housework), or perhaps at more irregular intervals (hedge cutting, window cleaning) and you need to consider whether some of the help needed can be supplied by family or friends. For example, you may consider asking for a professional carer to come in on weekdays while the family can provide cover at weekends and on bank holidays. This is very important because weekend and holiday cover is likely to be much more expensive and also because (you may be surprised to discover) the agency may simply not be able to provide cover at holiday times. It depends on how many of their staff are willing to work the 'unsocial hours'. Be aware of this because the agency will not necessarily tell you this in advance of your entering into a contract with them, although a good agency will make their provision clear in advance.

****

The agency we used said that they could cover 365 days of the year if we required it. But when our usual 'days' occurred over holiday time we had to re-book ahead to say that we wanted cover then. In addition we occasionally got letters to say that they actually could not provide cover on certain days. For example, one year when we had planned to go out on Boxing Day we received an apologetic letter just before Christmas saying that they couldn't provide cover that day so we had to change our plans at the last minute.

****

Discuss how the care will be provided: The agency may try to en-sure in so far as it is possible that it is always the same person who provides care and that someone else will only be sent in cases of sickness and holiday. They may, however, not be able to agree to this. They may have part-time workers and shift work-ers and job-share workers and the person coming to provide care may be different on different days and at different times. This is especially likely if the person you care for needs care at different times of the day – for example, in the morning with getting out of bed and dressed and in the evening with getting undressed and back into bed. Some elderly people, whilst accepting the need for regular help, will be upset with the seemingly impersonal nature of this type of provision. If the person you care for suffers from dementia, s/he may be afraid of strangers and bewildered by different carers appearing at different times and you would have to take this into consideration.

Find out what the carer will do: It has already been mentioned that some agencies only deal with one aspect of care. Even when agencies say that they will tackle multiple tasks, you need to clarify what is not allowed. For example, a carer may be allowed to give medicine provided you have left it out with the correct dosage (say, two pills in a container to be taken at midday) but may not be permitted to decide for themselves when to give a dose. Medicine is a difficult area. Some agencies will say that their carers can 'encourage' the person in their care to take medicine but not actually hand it to them. Similarly a carer may be prepared to heat up a ready meal but not to cook food from scratch. You will also have to bear in mind the time factor. Only so much can be achieved in a set amount of time. In one hour a carer could heat up a meal, wash up and quickly dust around but they couldn't also vacuum the house and make the bed. Usually the agency will give you guidance on this. Different agencies also have different rules about whether carers can take charge of money to buy shopping, for example. Most have a rule that carers cannot accept ex-gratia payments.

Check up on administrative details: All agencies must produce a statement of purpose and a service user's guide which details at the minimum:

- The aims and objectives of the agency and the type of services provided, including specialist services
- The people for whom the service is provided
- An overview of the process for the delivery of care and support
- Key contract terms and conditions: whether you will be issued with a contract by the agency and what arrangements have to be made for unusual occurrences
- The complaints procedure
- The Quality Assurance process
- Specific information on key policies and procedures. For example, you would want to ask whether, if the person

you care for goes on holiday or into hospital, a 'retainer' needs to be paid to the agency

- How to contact the Care Quality Commission (CQC), social services, health care authorities and the General Social Services Council (GSCC)
- The hours of operation and details of insurance cover.

This is the time to find out whether you or the person you care for will be invoiced and how often. If you have power of attorney you should specify that all invoices come to you. You should also ask about written care plans, and whether notes are left by the carer on each visit. Don't be misled into believing that an ultra-efficient administrative package means that the care is better or alternatively that late invoices mean a bad standard of care. The administration and the caring usually rest with two different departments of the agency and efficiency in one may not necessarily mean the best service in the other.

What to expect from the agency

After making initial contact and establishing that you want to take things further with the agency, the next step will be a visit by a care manager. If you employ a care worker from an agency without having an assessment by the council, the agency must carry out a full assessment of your care needs. At this visit they may also carry out what is known as a 'risk assessment' on your cared-for's home and circumstances. Even though professional carers carry out some tasks which other people find distasteful, or difficult, there are certain rules about what they are allowed to do, and the agency still has a duty regarding health and safety towards their employees. The care manager will want to look around the home and note unsafe equipment or problems which might prevent the carer giving the required service. They will also want to talk to the person concerned about the service s/he is going to receive. Only after this visit, and after receiving and signing the care agency contract, will you be able to arrange a date for the professional carers to begin visiting the person you care for.

All this can take some time – several weeks perhaps – and if social services are being involved it might take even longer. This is why you need to think about the need for professional care well in advance if you can. Also, once you have a system of care set up, you may be surprised to find that to extend or improve the care plan may, again, take time. It is not simply a matter of calling the care agency and saying that now you would like the carer to call three times a week instead of twice. Agencies have their rotas to arrange and are often short of staff prepared to do the tasks required. Again it is worth trying to foresee what might be needed a few months down the line and planning for it early on.

If you are employing the agency directly, you should be provided with a written contract within seven days of the start of the service. The agency must have a confidentiality policy, which they must provide to the client (you or the person you care for) and which must detail how they will hold and use personal data. There must also be clear, written policies and procedures covering how staff administer and assist with medication.

Even if you or the person you care for have arranged private care without involving social services you will not always be allowed to retain that privacy. Nearly all care agencies have strong links with the local authority social services departments and can and do report to these departments about individual clients if they think it necessary. If a case is reported to them, the local social services have what is known as a 'duty of care' and must make further enquiries.

****

We had begun to think that Mum needed further care from the agency on a daily basis and had arranged a family meeting to discuss this. The day before the meeting I was astonished to be called by the social services department who told me that the agency had reported to them that they were concerned about my mother's care and that they wished to set up a meeting with me. I was amazed that the agency had approached social services without talking to one of us first, but when I took this up with the Care Manager she was quite unapologetic and refused to accept that her behaviour was at all improper. To make matters worse, when we did agree the need for daily care the same agency then said they didn't have enough staff to provide it!

****

Once you have set things up with the care agency your day-to-day relationship, and that of the person you care for, will then be with the carer or carers who provide the actual services you have negotiated. It goes without saying that individual carers vary in how willing they are to go 'beyond the call of duty', and also in how well they manage to get on with your relative or friend. It is a good idea to have written a list of what you want the carer to do, whether on a daily or an occasional basis. For example, if you expect the carer to provide a lunchtime meal and to make the bed each day but you also require a variety of jobs (say, wiping out the fridge, vacuuming one room, cleaning the bathroom) on a regular, but not daily, basis it is best to ensure that a list is made, agreed to and kept available. Then, if your regular carer is replaced by someone else due to sickness or holiday, the replacement carer knows just what to do on any given day.

****

The first carer my mother-in-law had was absolutely wonderful. She carried out all the tasks we gave her and filled in her allotted time by doing odd jobs like tidying the freezer or polishing the bookshelves. She got on well with mother-in-law as well. One day when my mother-in-law had an acute attack of her arthritis and was unable even to get out of her chair to answer the door, the carer climbed into the house through a window to look after her! Unfortunately this carer had to retire due to illness, and although the next carer was pleasant and did what we wanted, she made it plain that she couldn't be expected to do anything extra.

****

If the person you care for dislikes having a professional carer, is a little awkward or suffers from dementia, then you may find there is a problem when the carer needs to gain entry to the house. Your relative/friend may refuse to answer the door, or may turn the carer away. Generally, this means that you (as the main contact) will be telephoned. Perhaps you will have to go round to the house to persuade your relative/friend to let the carer in. On the other hand, where the carer works to a strict schedule with other clients to visit, the visit on that day may have to be cancelled. Agencies vary in their attitude to these episodes. Some may not charge you, but others will maintain that their employee was ready and willing to do the agreed service and that payment must be made regardless. Not all professional carers are prepared to hold a front door key, but most are happy to take a key from a coded 'keysafe' outside the building and to let themselves in. You may need to resort to this if the person you care for needs help in getting out of bed.

Both the actual carers and the caring agency are usually used to awkward clients, to elderly people who are perhaps grumpy and difficult, and to clients suffering from dementia. They will often work hard to maintain their relationship with the client and the family in difficult circumstances. However, most professional carers have a schedule to keep and agencies have a business to run. It is important to understand their point of view when it comes to difficulties with the person you care for. However, the agency will have policies about certain things and you or the person you care for are at liberty to ask them about these in relation to such things as knocking/ringing the bell and speaking out before entering the home, who keeps a set of keys and where they are kept, the confidentiality of entry codes if you use a key safe, for example, and what alternative arrangements they have for gaining entry if the usual arrangements fall down, securing the house when they leave it and what they will do if your relative/friend has an accident.

Generally, the care agency will provide a timesheet or 'log' which the professional carer will complete on each visit. This is a very valuable piece of information for you since it will inform you about such matters as what your relative/friend has been given to eat, how s/he appeared physically to the carer, what work the carer has carried out and any problems which the carer wishes to bring to your attention. Where you have been forced to engage a professional carer because you are prevented yourself (perhaps because you have a job or you live at a distance) from seeing the person you care for on a daily basis, the log provides a useful tool for keeping in touch. You can also compare the daily log with the care plan which has been provided by the agency and point out any problems or potential difficulties early on.

If you do encounter any problems, then obviously the first thing to do is to raise them with the agency manager, or the care manager who deals with the person you care for. Then follow the agency's own complaints procedure. If the person you care for has dementia, or is muddled in her/his mind, then make absolutely sure of your facts first. You can try following the tips in Chapter 7, Dealing with dementia, in order to establish the truth as nearly as you can.

There are two elements here which are sometimes difficult to reconcile. You want the person you care for to be treated with care and concern for her/his dignity, and the agency carer is in a position of power if the person concerned is weak or helpless or unable to communicate. On the other hand, as pointed out in Chapter 7, sufferers may 'confabulate', or fill in memory gaps, with statements of what they think happened. However, it must be said that if you or the person you care for has real doubts about the care they are receiving, it may be better to switch to another agency if there is one available.

Help through the NHS

In some cases, and usually in emergencies, caring teams are also provided through the NHS. The work these teams do is sometimes referred to as **'reablement'**, or **'intermediate care'**. The name varies depending upon which area you live in. The reablement team can provide care up to three times per day for a limited period in the case of a 'crisis at home'. This means, for example, if the person you care for needs this level of care but you or s/he is unable to arrange your own provision immediately. It might apply if your relative or friend was being discharged from hospital following an accident or illness, or if the usual carer was ill and unable to supply the current level of care. The team is also able to cover some 'night sitting' if the person you care for is unable to be left alone all night. These teams consist of multi-disciplinary support workers trained for up to one year in various areas of caring, and the standard of care given is generally excellent. The teams are accessible via the district nursing team, the hospital from which discharge is being arranged, or social services; the needs of your relative/friend may be referred through any of these depending on circumstances. Unfortunately it is true to say that this help is not always offered as a matter of course when required, so be prepared to ask for it if you need it and to be gently insistent about your need. Also be aware that this kind of help is not always provided free of charge and the person you care for may have to contribute towards the cost.

Chapter 10

Managing change

My mother had a lot of trouble getting up from the sitting position due to a bad hip. It would take her ages to get up out of her chair if the doorbell rang or if she needed something from the next room. I could see that a 'riser/recliner' chair would be a real boon to her, but she refused to buy one even though she could afford it. In the end the family clubbed together and bought it as a birthday gift. Even then she resisted putting it in the sitting room where her usual chair was placed. Eventually, we installed the chair and showed her how to use it. At first she wouldn't use the mechanism, insisting on dragging herself up as before. Finally, my brother got quite cross with her and insisted that she use it. Within a week she was proclaiming to all and sundry what a marvellous invention it was!

****

Changes are hard for many of us and one of the biggest difficulties you may encounter whilst acting as carer may be trying to get your elderly relative or friend to change anything – routines, furniture, habitation – with which they are familiar. Even those who do not suffer from dementia may resist change. It takes some elderly people longer than others to come to terms with a new idea. An elderly person in the early stage of dementia may actually find any change in routine quite frightening.

This means it is important first to decide whether a change is really necessary. Often it can appear that a new way of doing things, a new piece of equipment, a move to new living accommodation, or an alteration in routine would be of benefit to the person we care for and we take it for granted that they will feel the same way about it. However, elderly people need familiar things and faces around them and may regard new people in their life, new items of furniture and especially new routines with suspicion. Even when something new would make life easier for them they may resist. It is easy to become very impatient with this type of resistance. If you want to introduce any change consider it in three steps:

- Is the change actually necessary or just convenient?
- Can smaller alterations or adjustments be made to prevent the need (or put off the need) for a major change?
- How can any necessary change be introduced in the least challenging way?

Moving home

Necessary or just convenient?

It often seems obvious to carers that their relative/friend's home is inconvenient and difficult to manage for someone less mobile than they used to be (and perhaps even a bit infirm). The inclination is to suggest a move – to a bungalow, a smaller house, a warden-managed complex, or a care home. It may be hard to understand the outright resistance such a suggestion often provokes. But it is the very familiarity of the living space which provides reassurance to the elderly person. They automatically know where every handhold is as they move from room to room. Their belongings are all stowed in familiar places so that they need scarcely think to carry out their everyday tasks. They may already have made small adaptations – moving a rug so that it doesn't cause them to trip, using an extension cord to make a power point easier to reach, adding a lower shelf in the bathroom – in the past to make their environment more convenient. Many elderly people have also gone to great lengths to make their home secure, installing door and window locks, for example, or a door chain, and they feel secure and relaxed indoors and in their own garden. Naturally they are resistant to the very idea of leaving these familiar surroundings. All this is quite apart from the simple fact that a widow or widower may have many happy memories of times spent with their partner and family in the house or flat where they may have lived together for many years. To move may seem like leaving the partner behind, even more than the loss due to death.

It is well documented that many elderly people who are forced to move home go from being quite self-sufficient and managing well around the house to needing help and being unable to cope. In part this is due to the unfamiliarity of the new home and to the loss of the sense of security which the elderly person previously had.

Can small adjustments prevent major change?

First, examine the present environment. Through social services or through the district nursing team you can ask for and arrange an occupational therapy (OT) assessment of your cared-for's home to plan where small adjustments can make the environment safer and more comfortable. The therapists will advise about such things as ramps to outside doors, grab rails, raised toilet seats, non-slip rugs, bathing aids and so on. Usually the person you care for, or the immediate family, will be expected to make the actual arrangements for these changes and to pay for them, although some items (raised toilet seats, for example) can be given on loan. The OT assessors will produce a written plan for any changes and agree with the person you care for (and you if you are present) on how the changes might be implemented and who is responsible for the implementation. If your relative or friend has suffered an illness or accident and spent some time in hospital, then s/he will not normally be sent home from hospital until an assessment of the home environment has been conducted to see if s/he can manage alone at home.

****

After Mum died we were appalled to discover the extent to which Dad was unable to manage. Mum had been helping him so much that we had not realised how difficult he found it to get up and down from a chair, to pull plugs out of the wall sockets and even to do things like opening food cans. My sister and I thought that a care home was the only answer but the GP arranged an OT assessment of the house for us. The OT assessor showed us how a number of quite minor things, like an electric can opener and some special grips for the taps and electric plugs, could make a huge difference. Of course Dad wanted to carry on living at home as long as he could, so luckily he made a big effort to learn to use all the 'aids'.

****

Some simple changes such as those mentioned above may make your relative/friend's life at home safer and more convenient. It may also give you, the carer, a little more peace of mind. From a safety point of view, a number of small changes can make the home more secure. Good door locks and a chain and spy-hole are the first essentials, though the chain should be used only to answer the door, not left on, in case someone needs to gain entrance in an emergency. The person you care for should be persuaded always to use the door chain if s/he does not know who the caller is. It is worth making a point not to let anyone into the house unless they are known to her/him. Bona fide traders will carry identification, but this is possible to imitate. An easily purchased and fitted closed-circuit TV camera by the front door may give you and your relative/friend some peace of mind. These are obtainable from DIY stores and can be attached to the normal television for viewing who is at the door. They take only a few moments to fit and this can be done by anyone reasonably competent at DIY.

Introducing necessary major changes in the least challenging way

If a house move is really vital then you will need to approach things slowly. This is something for the whole family to discuss and consider. Strangely what often happens is that all the family talk around a solution and forget to include the elderly relative or friend in question in their discussions! Remember that it is the elderly person and her/his needs which are being discussed as well as the convenience of the carers. You should ask the person you care for what her/his preferences are. S/he may be adamant about wanting to stay in her/his own house. It will take time and patience to convince her/him otherwise. It may help to take all the alternatives and discuss them one by one, pointing out the pros and cons and explaining the possibilities.

- Moving in with family or friends – consider the following: is there room available in the home of any of the family? Are the family prepared to make any changes necessary in their household? How would privacy issues be managed? What financial contribution would your relative or friend make to the household? What would be the effect on other members of the household?
- Living alone – consider the following: can a suitable house, bungalow or flat be found near to one or other family member so that visitors can drop in and perhaps grandchildren be taken to visit? Does your relative/friend need to have help on hand in case of emergency (warden-

managed accommodation)? Can help be arranged for tasks which are too difficult (professional carers or family members and friends)?

- Moving to a communal residential home – Few elderly people look forward to the idea of giving up their independence in this way. It will take time and much discussion to persuade your elderly relative or friend that this is the right move. Consider what type of accommodation is necessary. How much can your relative/friend afford in fees? In what area should you look for a home? (For further useful discussion see Chapter 11 on Care and nursing homes.)

Getting out and about

If your elderly relative or friend has always been driven or accompanied by their partner – or driven her/himself and is no longer fit to do so – s/he may resist the very idea of taking buses or taxis and expect you or some other member of the family to carry out the job of chauffeur and companion as her/his partner did. You may be prepared to do this, but it will still involve some changes in routine.

Can small adjustments prevent major change?

You may only need to help your relative/friend to gain confidence in going out alone. Otherwise, you may need to give some very active help in the way of applying for bus passes, writing down taxi service telephone numbers and initially accompanying her/him on the bus or in the taxi until these new modes of travel are familiar.

Introducing the change in the least challenging way

Try to give full attention to the details which may make the person you care for reluctant to use these services. For example, elderly people may not like waiting at bus stops alone because they are afraid of being attacked and 'mugged'. They may feel awkward getting in and out of taxis if they are a little disabled or they may feel that they do not know how much to tip the taxi driver. If driving the person you care for around regularly is likely to cause you severe inconvenience, then it is worth persevering in trying to overcome these objections. You might, for example, suggest that s/he teams up with a neighbour for trips on the bus. You might investigate whether there is a local taxi service which specialises in helping the elderly (see Chapter 3 on Getting about).

You may consider that the person you care for would be helped by using a walking aid long before s/he accepts the idea. Use of a simple walking stick may not be resisted much, but to many the notion of using a 'Zimmer frame' is totally unacceptable. Fortunately there are many modern wheeled walking aids available now which may be found more acceptable (see Chapter 3). Your relative or friend should be the one who chooses the walking aid and there are many shops and mobility centres where you can take her/him to try out different styles and designs. Ask the district nurse where would be the best place for you to go locally to look at walking aids. The district nurse may suggest that your elderly relative or friend, has a physiotherapy assessment to decide the most suitable frame or trolley. It may help to persuade a reluctant user if it is suggested that it can at first just be used 'now and again'. Once they are used to the mobility and stability which these aids give, most users are enthusiasts and recommend them to friends.

New furniture and fittings

Necessary or just convenient?

Buying new furniture to replace that which has grown shabby is just convenient. Replacing items which are damaged and might cause accidents (electric fires, cookers, worn rugs etc) is necessary. A newer and better washing machine might just be convenient. A microwave might be necessary. The most difficult step will probably be to persuade the person you care for to accept the new items, but people differ in this as in everything else.

****

After my mother had her stroke she was so keen not to be a burden that she immediately asked me to order her meals-on-wheels and to arrange the purchase of a walker trolley so that she would be allowed home. My mother-in-law on the other hand refused even to accept a helping hand to get in and out of the car and could never be brought to see that in refusing help of any kind she placed more of a burden on all of us.

****

Can small adjustments prevent major change?

Consider whether clearer instructions would help someone use the equipment they already own more easily. User instructions can be scanned into a computer and reprinted in larger print, for example. Could moving the furniture or equipment make it easier to use? Perhaps an extension cord would facilitate this. Would a larger kitchen bin mean fewer trips out to the dustbin? Would adding more table lamps save moving a favourite chair into a different position? Would a grab rail mean there was no need for a raised toilet seat?

Introducing the change in the least challenging way

Remember that it is not you who is going to use the furniture or the equipment every day; it is your elderly relative or friend.

Discuss with her/him whether a particular appliance or piece of equipment would make life easier. Expect reluctance to agree and take the time to talk through the reasons why a particular item might help, stressing that it will allow her/him to remain independent. Many people are converted to an idea after they have seen how it makes life easier for a friend or neighbour, so if you can show her/him, say, the way that 'old Mrs So-and-so down the road gets about with her walker trolley' it might be a real advantage. You could collect a few catalogues and take time to look through them to see which particular types of equipment might be most useful. Disability Centres and shops welcome visitors and here you will be able to touch and try out different equipment or to see it demonstrated.

Once the person you care for is in possession of the appliance or piece of equipment, make sure that s/he knows how to use it. For major items such as a stairlift, the suppliers will often include a familiarisation session as part of the supply package, but you may still need to ensure that your relative or friend uses the equipment on a daily basis and does not forget instructions for use. For some items (a rising/reclining chair with an electric motor, for example) you may find that you need to go over the methods of use several times before your relative or friend is confident in its use.

If you are arranging for a new appliance (such as a microwave oven) which your elderly relative or friend may not be familiar with, then you will need to take some time to demonstrate how it can be used and to stress safety measures for use. If a family member is competent on a computer, s/he can scan direction leaflets and print them out in large print. Alternatively, you might reduce the instructions to their most basic and copy these out and leave them in a prominent place near the equipment. As an example, if your elderly relative or friend acquires an automatic washing machine and will only be likely to use one or two programmes, write out clearly the instructions for these and tape them to the machine.

None of the above is meant to imply that the person you care for is too stupid to understand instructions. Indeed, many elderly people will take a delight in learning to use all the functions of a piece of equipment and get full use from it. Others with perhaps poor sight or poor concentration will find that the above measures make life easier for them.

Help in the house

Necessary or just convenient?

Can the person you are caring for manage all that is necessary even if it takes her/him a little longer than it might take you? Can you or another family member undertake to do what s/he can't manage without too much inconvenience or difficulty?

Can small adjustments prevent major change?

Small adjustments can range from a little occasional part-time help with difficult jobs, such as gardening or window cleaning, to visits on a regular basis for set jobs. Elderly people are often quite amenable to having someone help with the 'heavy' cleaning and if it is a simple cleaning service that is needed, this is best obtained by advertising locally or using a cleaning agency. The agencies are much more expensive, but you and your relative or friend have the benefit of knowing that the cleaning staff have had their references checked and have a reputation to maintain with the agency. It may not be very difficult to persuade the person you care for that s/he needs extra help in the house, but some people feel that having 'a stranger' coming into their house is an invasion of their privacy. They may try to convince you that they can manage by themselves or may ask you to help them instead. A lot of gentle persuasion may be needed. It might help to go through tasks with your relative or friend and try to start in a small way. Perhaps someone could come in just to trim the hedges to start with, or just to clean the windows once a month. This 'toe in the water' approach may then make the person you care for more amenable to extend the help. On the other hand, you may have to be quite firm in pointing out that your own time is limited if this is the case and that your relative or friend will have to begin to trust others for some of these tasks. Unless s/he is on a very low income, there is unlikely to be any free help available and it may be that you and s/he will have to settle for the amount of help that can be afforded.

It is quite important when organising help in the house to go through the tasks which you and the person you care for require to be done and to specify how frequently. You may be surprised to discover that some cleaners 'don't do beds' or that others consider cleaning and defrosting the fridge to be outside their duties, for example. If you are considering using an agency, then it helps to make careful enquiries in the first telephone call. Some specify that they only handle 'light housework' which is the area your relative/friend can probably manage themselves. It is the heavier work where help is most often needed, such as vacuuming under beds, cleaning windows and ovens, and mowing the lawn. Other help agencies specialise in offering companionship, running small errands and doing light shopping but do not offer cleaning services at all. Make a list of the tasks that need doing. Make a shortlist of likely agencies or private cleaners. Then telephone each and ask first if they or their staff will undertake these tasks before entering into enquiries about prices or availability. This will save a good deal of time in the long run.

****

My mother and father had had the services of a cleaner once a week for a few years. Gradually on my visits I began to notice that some things were not as clean as they could be and that the bedclothes were changed very infrequently. I asked them why the cleaner wasn't doing the work but they always prevaricated.

Eventually I asked the cleaner directly. She told me then that she 'didn't do beds or bathrooms' and that this had been understood by my parents when they employed her. But of course, as they grew more frail, they were unable to do these things themselves. They liked the woman and did not want to upset her or lose her services. In the end the solution was to employ a second cleaner to do the things the first one wouldn't do!

****

Introducing the change in the least challenging way

Accepting help with personal care is one of the biggest challenges that may face you and the person you care for. Many people need help as they grow older with dressing, washing and toileting due to disability from arthritis or other disabling conditions, and people with dementia need help in these areas because they become unable to begin or to carry through simple everyday personal care. Most of us very much dislike the idea of having help with personal care and your elderly relative or friend may disguise her/his need for such help as long as possible. Some people will insist that they need help from you, especially if you are a relative, and not from an outsider even when they know you are unable to provide it due to other commitments.

****

My mother needed help to get in and out of bed after her stroke. She also needed some help with fastenings and things like that when dressing. However, she was quite capable of managing to use the toilet and of washing and showering herself. For ages she refused to tell us that she needed any help because she was terrified that any carer would insist on helping her to wash or shower. Once we discovered what worried her we were able to arrange for a carer to come in the morning and evening but gave them strict instructions to let Mum wash herself and use the toilet in privacy. For the first week one of us visited when the carer came to ensure that our instructions were carried out. This gave Mum confidence and she accepted the help she needed.

****

On the other hand, some people would prefer to accept such help from professionals rather than from a relative or friend. It might help to point out that those who provide personal care choose to do it because they like helping others, that they are specially trained, and that they are used to the tasks which your relative or friend might find embarrassing. It will certainly help if you allow the person you care for to get used to the idea gradually, to help in selecting the provider and to give a clear idea of what help they want and need and what they can manage for themselves. Here again there are many items of equipment available to help those with minor disabilities to remain independent for as long as possible (see Chapter 1 on aids and equipment).

Summing up

Managing change will be more successful if you apply the above simple principles. Change management entails thoughtful planning and sensitive implementation, and above all, consultation with, and involvement of, the people affected by the changes. If you force change on people, especially elderly people, difficult problems can arise.

In all cases of necessary change, be prepared to be patient, to involve the person you care for in decisions and to allow her/him to talk, to voice any fears and worries beforehand. Where someone suffers from dementia, or where not making the changes would endanger the safety of your relative or friend, it may be necessary to be firm and even to overrule her/him, but where at all possible it will pay to introduce changes slowly and cautiously.

Chapter 11

Choosing a care home or nursing home

The question is bound to arise eventually – has the time come when it would be more appropriate for your elderly relative or friend to move into an environment where a higher level of care would be available? Many people have to make a decision about a care home in a crisis, perhaps after a fall or an illness, or the death of a partner. Looking back they often wish they'd had longer to look around. So if you think the person you care for might need a care home in the future, it's a good idea to do some planning sooner rather than later. This would also give your loved one time to get used to the idea. This may be much easier for her/him if initially the suggestion is put forward simply as something that 'might happen sometime in the future'. You may find it useful to refer to Chapter 10 on Managing change when you and the person you care for tackle the task of moving into a residential home.

If the person you care for lives alone, then you and s/he may begin to feel that there is a need for a more constant presence as a back-up. If you are already living with your relative or friend and providing live-in care, then it may be that you feel you can no longer cope or are no longer able to provide the level of care required. You may consider the possibility of your relative or friend moving into warden-supported accommodation. However, you do need to be aware that in most accommodation of this kind the warden is supposed to be there in case of emergency only. In some types of complexes the warden may, as a matter of goodwill, also run small errands for the residents and carry out small services for them, but in others there is strict 'call service' operating, which means that unless the person you care for actually calls for help (or in some cases fails to answer the routine check-up telephone call that the warden makes) no follow-up will be made. If you are afraid that the person you care for may simply need help in an emergency (perhaps following a fall) then this may be sufficient for your purposes. However, for most of us the big change comes when we, and others, have to consider the need for accommodation where help is always on hand as and when required.

Types of residential accommodation

Residential accommodation for the elderly falls into three categories. There are 'care homes', 'nursing homes' and 'dual care homes' (care and nursing). There are also homes that specialise in caring for people with dementia. The person you care for may need one type of accommodation now and to move on to another later in life.

Care homes

Care homes are the ones we tend to think of as 'old people's homes'. This accommodation is meant for elderly, reasonably fit people who can look after themselves to a certain extent in everyday matters. These homes are not meant for elderly people who need 'nursing care'. If the person you care for were to live in this type of home, s/he would have a room or apartment which would probably be cleaned for her/him, and communal lounges and other facilities would be provided. Meals would also be provided, probably in a communal dining room (although some homes provide a kind of 'room service' for meals). The benefit of this type of home is that the burden of providing for everyday living in the form of cooking, cleaning and associated shopping is lifted from the residents, they have company should they wish for it and help is at hand if an emergency arises. Many such homes provide social activities on site and such useful facilities as a visiting library, film service, and small shop for necessities such as toiletries or stamps. These homes do not provide for elderly people who need nursing care every day, although some may have a visiting doctor or nursing service. Usually these homes can provide some help with personal care if your relative or friend needs help with washing and dressing.

Nursing homes

Nursing homes are a separate category of home. They have a trained nurse on hand at all times and they will provide for people who are less able to manage their own personal care. They are also able to provide nursing for chronic conditions such as leg ulcers, pressure sores and certain disabilities and conditions (for example, diabetes) where the intervention of a nurse might be required periodically. Different staff in these homes will deal not only with routine cleaning and domestic chores (as in a care home) but will also provide help with washing, dressing, moving about, and eating and drinking if required.

Dual registered homes

Dual registered homes offer both residential and nursing care. They may be the right choice if you think the level of care your relative or friend needs may change in the future, or for couples who each need different levels of care. Dual registered homes will normally be registered for specific numbers of nursing beds and residential beds, and availability will depend upon the home's assessment of your relative or friend's needs and the availability of an appropriate bed. It is possible to find registered homes where all the types of care are provided in different buildings on the same site, so that if your relative or friend starts off needing simple nursing care but later suffers from dementia, for example, s/he can simply move to another building with the minimum of disruption.

Homes caring for those with dementia

These specialist homes provide for those elderly who are mentally infirm (usually dementia sufferers) and who may or may not be able to manage some of their own personal care, but who in any case need a close level of supervision, either to stop them getting lost and confused, or to prevent them harming themselves, or to help them with everyday living. Some residential care homes and some nursing homes also offer places to a limited number of people with dementia.

Paying for residential care

The state only provides free residential care for the least well off. It is therefore quite likely that your relative or friend will have to pay at least some of the costs of accommodation and personal care in a residential or nursing home. The amount the state (actually the local authority of the area in which your friend or relative lives) pays depends upon the income and capital that person has. The capital amount taken into consideration is different in England, Scotland and Wales. If the person you care for has income and capital below a set amount, then the state will fund the full cost of residential accommodation. Some payment will be made if her/his income and capital are above the minimum, up to a maximum. If s/he has capital over this maximum, s/he will have to pay the full cost of accommodation. If her/his income and capital fall below the upper amount whilst s/he is in a care home, then s/he will become eligible for help from the state. If your friend or relative wants a more expensive home than the local authority is willing to pay for, you are allowed to arrange a 'third party contribution' (often known as top-up fees) from another source. The full value of your relative or friend's personal home would be included in her/his assets only if s/he lives alone. In addition, the local authority will disregard the value of the person's home for 12 weeks after her/his admission to permanent nursing or residential care. This will mean that if, without the house, the value of the person's accountable assets falls below the threshold s/he will have a breathing space to make plans, or sell the house. The person you care for will be expected to use all their income – including any pension, benefits, and so on – to fund care. However, a small weekly amount can be kept as spending money.

Nursing care is defined as care that must be provided by a registered nurse. An assessment needs to be done to see whether this level of care is needed. If it is, it will be funded by the state. The payment depends on whether nursing needs are assessed as low, medium or high. This contribution applies whether care is funded privately or by the local authority. If the person you care for is paying his/her own fees, s/he will still have to pay for accommodation and personal care (such as help with dressing or bathing). Quite often the individual nursing home will help you to make the claim for nursing care contributions and once you and your relative or friend have decided on a home, then it is worth you discussing this with the administrative staff there.

The rules for funding are quite complicated and are in the process of being fundamentally changed. They do differ depending upon the individual local authority. It is important to consult local and up-to-date guidance to obtain accurate information.

****

My mother was already in receipt of an attendance allowance. Once we had settled on a nursing home I thought I would have to go through a lot more form-filling to try to claim nursing fees but the matron of the home told me that she would attend to that. Apparently 'nursing care needs' cover a variety of things. For example, the fact that my mother had a pressure sore meant that she qualified for some nursing. I was really glad to be able to let the staff at the home deal with the claim for us.

****

Paying for care is a complex subject, and everyone's situation is different. You should seek advice about your relative or friend's individual case. Organisations which offer specialist advice are listed at the end of the book. Immediate care insurance may be suitable if you are currently considering helping the person you care for to move into a care home. It involves paying a single large sum at the time you and s/he decide residential care is needed. The cost is based on the length of time the insurer thinks care will be needed, and the level of care required. While the cost can seem a large amount, it should provide a fixed payment for as long as your friend or relative needs care, and can protect the rest of her/his assets. The payments are tax-free if they are generally made directly to a care home and are portable if you and your relative or friend decide to move to a different home. Further information on this subject can be found in Chapter 2 on Financial matters.

Drawing up a short list

You and the person you care for will wish to take time to research the availability of places and to view individual homes. To begin your search it may be useful to speak to people you know, for their recommendations, as well as your relative or friend's GP and/or the district nurse. Your local social services department should be able to provide a list of registered homes in your area; otherwise you could search the internet or research in the local telephone directory if this is still available. A useful idea would be for you and your relative or friend (and any other members of the family who might be involved) to first make a list of any criteria which are important to you. For example, you might want a home which is near enough for you to visit frequently. Your relative or friend might have her/his own ideas about room sizes, the standard of common facilities (dining room, lounge) or the availability of en-suite toilet and bathing facilities. Perhaps s/he enjoys being outdoors and the size and type of grounds are a consideration.

****

When we started looking for a residential nursing home, my mother-in-law was already suffering from dementia and unable to make a decision about where she wanted to live. We were looking locally, and because she had been a keen gardener we were zeroing in on places with pleasant communal gardens. But in the event my sister-in-law decided that she wanted her mother to live nearer to where she lived and she did her own research, eventually finding a really nice nursing home two hours away from where we lived. It seemed strange not to be able to visit as frequently as we had been used to, but we had to agree that the nursing home chosen was just right.

****

Every residential home, whether run by the local authority or privately, is overseen by the Care Quality Commission (CQC). Registration of the home is subject to certain standards and these are the criteria which govern each inspection. After the annual inspection a report is made, and these reports are lodged in the local public library. Many homes also publish the results of the report on their website if they have one, and some local authorities may publish these reports on their website too. The report includes information on the number of beds, the immediate surrounding area, the number and qualifications of the staff and the facilities provided. It also includes the fee rates. Once you have produced a list of homes to consider, then the annual report is probably a good place to start to reduce your list to a shortlist of places you and the person you care for would like to view. However, it is useful to bear in mind that a CQC rating takes into account a range of details which you may not necessarily consider important for your friend or relative. For example, the CQC rating may be reduced if staff records are not maintained in good order.

If the person you care for will be paying all the care home's fees, you and s/he can contact homes directly. Once you have found a home you like, the home will make an assessment of your relative or friend's needs, so that they can be sure they can offer the right kind of care. If your relative or friend needs nursing care, for example, the home will have to be able to supply this.

If the local authority is being asked to help with all or part of the fees, you should speak first to your relative or friend's GP and the local social services department. They will carry out an assessment of your needs, and produce a report called a care plan that outlines the care, including any nursing care, they think is needed. If your local authority is assisting with funding, it doesn't mean you have to choose one of their homes. You can still do your own research locally and you can request any home that accepts residents funded by the local authority. However, the local authority will want to be sure that the home is suitable for your relative or friend's needs and doesn't cost more than it would usually pay for that type of care. If a more expensive home is wanted than the authority is willing to pay for, you or the person you care for will be allowed to 'top up' the state contribution from another source. You may be surprised to know that the majority of care homes in the UK are owned by the independent sector, and that 70 per cent of residents have their fees paid partly or wholly by their local authority.

An initial telephone call to each home on your short list will help to clarify some points and to reduce the list still further. Simply assessing whether the phone is answered promptly, whether the person answering is helpful and assured, whether your questions are answered clearly and fully, and whether a visit is offered or further information (for example, referral to a website or an offer of a brochure) is provided, will help you to decide whether to follow up with a visit. Be wary if the person you speak to suggests that you only visit at a certain time or on a certain day. Of course you will want to time your visit for when the matron, manager or some other person with knowledge can be on hand to help you, but a well-run home should have nothing to hide from a chance visitor.

If the person you care for has some specific criteria of her/ his own when considering a care or nursing home, then in some respects you will have a ready-made short list of homes. If, for example, s/he is a Roman Catholic and wants a home run by a religious order, or, if Jewish, kosher cookery is important, or if s/he will not consider going into a home where pets are not allowed, then the choice will be restricted. The choice will also be restricted by the type of home required as detailed above. You choice might further be restricted by the scale of fees that the person you care for can afford, or which the local authority is prepared to pay. However, after taking these things into consideration you will probably have a list of three or four homes which you will wish to visit.

Taking a look – determining your criteria

What things you look for on your visit will depend upon the

wishes and circumstances of the person you care for. It is possible to obtain standard lists of 'things to look for' and 'questions to ask', but these will of course be generic in nature and it is more useful to decide about what the most important things are for your friend or relative personally, and then add on a wish list or a list of things s/he would be unwilling to accept in a new home. Listed below are some factors you might want to consider, and some suggestions as to how you can decide what fits your own and your relative or friend's particular criteria.

Locality

Is the home in the locality or community your relative or friend wants? S/he may want to be near to where you live (or another family member), or conveniently situated to visit friends or to have friends and family visit her/him. So the accessibility of the home may be very important: whether it is on a bus route, or near a railway station, or whether it has ample car parking. The person you care for may want to visit local amenities, such as shops, churches or pubs. If s/he has enjoyed a good social life, s/he will want to be able to continue this as far as possible, so s/he may, for example, want to be near the church s/he has been attending, the club s/he belongs to, or the shops s/he prefers to visit. S/he may want to live in a home where one or more of her/his friends already live(s).

Immediate surroundings

Most homes have some sort of garden, but you should consider the surroundings as carefully as you would if the person you care for were moving into a private home. For example, s/he may not want a home situated too near a busy and noisy main road, s/he may want to have good views of gardens and countryside from the windows, or alternatively s/he may want somewhere

where s/he can 'watch the world go about its business' even if s/he cannot go out much. In such a case, a home with windows looking onto the street might be preferred. If there is a communal garden, then what is it like? If the person you care for is, or has been, a keen gardener, s/he might think interesting shrubs and plants and the chance to help with some small garden tasks are more important than clipped grass and a tidy appearance. If s/he particularly enjoys being outside, then it is worth checking if it is easy to go out into the gardens and whether there are comfortable seats in the garden and smooth paths for walking. On your visit take time to notice if anyone is making use of the garden and whether staff encourage this. Most homes will tell you that anyone can go outside at will, but further questioning may elicit the response 'They only have to ask', or 'If the weather is suitable'. However, most people with dementia will not be able to ask to use the garden and, while the weather may be an important factor in garden use, who is to decide if the weather is too bad?

Accommodation

Remember that this is to be your relative or friend's home. Naturally the communal areas should be well decorated, bright and cheerful and clean. The home should smell fresh and there should be no unpleasant odours. It might be important to the person you care for that s/he can have her/his own room decorated to her/his own taste, so this is something you may want to check. You will also want to check if s/he can bring items of her/his own furniture if this is important to her/him, as well as pictures, ornaments and other items. Some homes allow pets and this may be a major criterion. Some homes will allow residents to bring their own curtains, rugs and bedding, and again this may be a very important factor. You should also check on some things that you may think would be taken for granted. For example, is it possible for the heating to be adjusted in different rooms, and can your relative or friend easily open and close the windows in her/his room? Everyone feels temperature differently and having control over his/her own 'microclimate' might be a major factor for your relative or friend. S/he might like to have her/his own telephone line and you can check whether this will be allowed, though mobile phones have made this less of an issue. Most homes are now happy for residents to have their own television in their room, but perhaps the person you care for prefers the radio or to listen to music? Or to find their entertainment on-line? You may want to see if the facilities would be available for this and whether residents have access to wi-fi.

****

The Matron of the home we were viewing had two rooms available. She was rather worried about showing us one of them, explaining that the occupant had recently died and had never been a very tidy person. She didn't want us to get the wrong impression from an untidy room. In fact I was more impressed that the previous occupant had been allowed to be untidy – in other words, at least her room was her personal space and she could relax in it in her own way. It was this respect for the individual that made us choose this home in the end.

****

Equipment

If the person you care for needs help with daily living, then you should pay special heed to the facilities available. There should be enough bathrooms and they should have proper toilet aids and items such as bath hoists, accessible showers and emergency call facilities. Many homes now offer en-suite toilet and washing facilities, and this may be a major factor for your relative or friend. Some people particularly dislike using communal washing and bathing areas. Some homes still offer shared rooms and this too may not suit the person you care for.

Most nursing homes have a call system in each room, but you may want to check if this is easy for your relative or friend to use, and perhaps see for yourself how quickly it is answered. If your relative or friend needs help to move around, you might want to check for handrails in passages and communal rooms and to see if rollator trolleys or walking frames are allowed, and if the passages and doorways are wide enough to accommodate them. If the person you care for particularly wants a ground-floor room because of difficulty using stairs, this may be a major factor on your checklist. Homes will naturally have stair-lifts, or elevators, where these are required, but your relative or friend may not be able or willing to use these on her/his own, and a room on an upper floor would therefore not suit at all.

Communal areas

You and your relative or friend may want to think about the security of the home. Although visiting should be allowed at any time, there should be a way of checking visitors in, and doors onto the street or non-enclosed gardens ought to be securely fastened to prevent undesirable or unauthorised people wandering into the home. The person you care for may be concerned about the security of her/his own possessions, so you may wish to query whether residents can lock their rooms when they leave them or whether there are facilities to secure cash and valuables.

Some homes have a dining room, but others serve residents' meals in their rooms or in the residents' communal lounge. Some offer a mix of both. You may want to enquire whether residents can choose where to eat and whether they can invite visitors to eat a meal with them, either in the dining room or in their own room provided notice is given. (Your relative or friend would expect to pay for any guests, of course.) Being able to invite guests for a meal may make all the difference to the acceptance of the idea of a residential home being really a 'home'.

Not all homes can offer two lounges, but the old-fashioned picture of a roomful of elderly people blankly gazing at a TV screen might fill you with horror. If there is only one lounge, then you might like to enquire whether the television is switched on continually, or how and when it is decided what will be viewed. Of course, the person you care for can always escape to her/ his own room, but not everyone wants to spend the day in one room. What other communal rooms are there? Is there a bar, for instance, or a games room, or a library? Which of these might be important to the person you care for? If being able to smoke (or choosing not to be exposed to other people's smoke) is important, then you will want to enquire about the smoking policy – that is, whether there are smoking and non-smoking areas and whether smoking is allowed in residents' rooms.

Facilities and entertainment

How important these are depends upon how active your relative or friend is, and how independent. If s/he enjoys an active social life in the community and intends to continue this, then s/ he may not be too concerned about 'in-house' entertainment. In this case, discuss and examine the ease with which residents can plan outings or opt out of meals, and whether any transport is organised by the home to get to local events. If your relative or friend is suffering from dementia, then some things, like music therapy or reminiscence memory therapy, say, might be more important than outings and films. So you would want to know whether these types of therapy are organised and what facilities are available to stimulate the minds of people with dementia.

If your relative or friend is mentally active but has physical problems in getting about, then the most important facilities might, for example, be visiting entertainment (films and live shows), library-book supplies, visits by hairdressers, facilities for people with hearing/visual difficulties, or availability of facilities to carry out any hobbies or interests.

****

Whilst viewing homes for my mother-in-law who suffered from dementia, my sister-in-law visited one home which made a great display of the many 'therapies' available. At first she was very impressed, but during the visit it became clear that residents were more or less forced to take part in the activities whether they wanted to or not, on the grounds that they were unable to decide for themselves what would be 'good for them'. My sister-in-law made a throwaway remark that the number of activities might leave the residents quite exhausted and received a very frosty response!

****

Some details about facilities need checking as a matter of course. For example, you could ask to see the laundry room and enquire whether laundry of personal belongings and bed linen is charged as extra. Sometimes room cleaning is also charged as extra, and you might like to enquire whether the rooms are cleaned on a daily or weekly basis. The person you care for may want to continue to be seen by her/his own GP and so you would want to check whether this is possible. Depending upon the area, it may be that your relative or friend's GP would not be able to visit. Similarly, it can be very useful to know what arrangements are made for visits by or to chiropodists, physiotherapists, opticians and dentists. Don't assume that there is a standard procedure.

Catering

If your friend or relative has special dietary needs, then, of course, this would be at the head of your list of questions. If religious dietary considerations are important (no meat on Friday and abstinence days, or kosher cooking, for example), then your choice of home might be limited. But even if this is not the case, you and the person you care for might like to know the standard of the cooking, whether a visitor can be invited to join a meal, what sort of choice of menu there is and whether meals must be taken in a particular room or in residents' own rooms if they wish. You could also enquire whether alcohol is allowed and can be ordered or bought for your friend or relative if this is important to her/him.

It could be worth organising your visit to coincide with a meal time to get your own ideas of the quality of food served, the serving arrangements, and the state of the food when it actually reaches the residents.

Staffing and daily concerns

The published inspection report should give details of staff qualifications. Some demands for training may seem excessive to you and you may be more concerned as to whether the staff seem kind and caring and whether other residents seem cheerful and calm in their presence. There are now rules about the number of staff who have to have received a certain level of training, but training does not guarantee kindness and consideration, nor does it ensure that those caring for your friend or relative will maintain her/his dignity and take extra trouble to accommodate individual wishes. It can be useful to enquire about the number of staff on duty, including those on duty at night. A nursing home should have a trained nurse on duty at all times. You may also like to make enquiries about the use of 'bank staff' and 'agency staff'. Most homes will have to make use of these at times of staff holiday or illness, but it will obviously be more pleasant for your relative or friend if s/he is generally looked after by the same people whom there will be a chance to get to know.

These days homes have a personal 'care plan' for each resident and you can enquire about these and ask whether you will be able to see the notes made about your relative or friend's care during your visits.

****

When my son and I visited the nursing home where my father eventually lived we had to wait for a short time in the hallway until the Matron was available to see us. We were sitting outside one of the rooms and the cleaner was working inside. What impressed me was the manner in which she chatted to the elderly lady whose room it was. The old lady was clearly unable to answer but the cleaner kept up a really pleasant and cheerful conversation and took such care when moving the old lady's possessions about that we gained a very good impression straightaway.

****

It is also useful to make enquiries about whether there are set times for getting up and going to bed and whether residents can request a bath or shower when it suits them. Of course, in a busy home some structure has to be maintained, but it could be very annoying for your friend or relative if s/he is always got out of bed first because her/his room is at the end of a particular corridor!

As already mentioned, you should enquire about the visiting policy and be very wary of homes where there is much restriction on visiting. The best homes allow visiting at any hour of the day or night, although of course they should monitor the admission of visitors. If the person you care for is active, s/he may want to help prepare meals or clean around the home or even arrange flowers and set tables etc. In this case, find out whether such help is welcomed. Not everyone wants to be waited on hand and foot.

Fees

Finally, you will want to make enquiries about payments. You should be careful to ascertain what is included in the standard weekly or monthly charge – for example, does the charge include laundry, chiropody or hairdressing? Some homes make an extra charge for toiletries such as soap and shampoo, or for extra drinks and refreshments. If extra charges are made for such items, when and how are they billed? Check how often fees are reviewed. It can be galling to be quoted a fee only for it to be increased within a month. It is easy to forget to ask such details as whether fees are payable in advance, whether they can be paid by direct debit and, especially, what happens to fees paid in advance if your relative or friend leaves the home mid-month or dies. If you hold power of attorney or otherwise manage your friend or relative's financial affairs, then you need to ensure that the bills will be sent directly to you.

After the move

My mother was suffering from mild dementia when she moved to a care home. I used to visit once a week and became a bit concerned because she said that they had stew for dinner every day. So I changed my routine and visited on several occasions around meal times. Of course, I found that the menu was good and varied. Because I had always visited on the same day and her memory was short, she could only remember what she had eaten that day. Sometimes it was goulash, sometimes curry, sometimes casseroled beef, but to her it was always 'stew'.

****

Chapter 11

Once your friend or relative is settled in the home, you will be able to plan your visits. Hopefully you have chosen a home which allows unrestricted visiting; it is a good idea to vary the times and days of your visits or to plan with other friends or family so that visits are spread over different days and times. It is always useful to see how the home runs at different times of the day and to get an idea of the routine. Visits are important for your relative or friend, who will look forward to seeing you and to the variation in her/his day. Visits are also important for you because they enable you to see how your friend or relative is cared for. In the early days, s/he may have several grumbles, but these are likely to be the result of settling in to a new home and a new routine. If you have serious worries about any aspect of care, or behaviour of the staff, always follow them up.

- Always listen carefully if the person you care for complains. If s/he suffers from dementia it is even more important to try to understand her/his concerns. (Some tips about unravelling confused speech are given in Chapter 7 on dementia.)
- Try if possible to get the name of the member or members of staff concerned.
- Always carry your concerns to the Matron or Care Home Manager in person.
- Ask for a follow-up interview to hear how your concerns have been addressed.
- Keep bringing your concerns forward even if you are treated as a nuisance. (Your relative or friend needs your help.)
- Keep written notes of any conversations you have about such concerns, making sure you write them up as soon as possible after they've taken place.
- If you are part of a family or group of friends try to maintain a united front when handling any concerns/ complaints.

****

I was my uncle's only visitor. One day he told me that the staff had dropped him on the floor when giving him a bath. He said that his leg hurt. When I asked the staff they denied that any accident had happened and suggested he was confused. To be honest I felt rather intimidated. Two years later he had some sort of scan done and the report said that there was evidence of an old injury, 'possibly a break in the limb'. I felt really guilty for not making more fuss at the time. But I felt even more angry at the apparent 'cover-up' by the staff at the home.

****

It is really important to continue to visit your relative or friend as often as you can, even if s/he suffers from dementia and appears not to be aware of your visit. It is an unfortunate fact that in some homes, those who are visited frequently and have relatives or friends to speak up for them are those who are best cared for. Although it is easy to blame care home staff for this, it is worth remembering that the homes are frequently short-staffed and staff are overworked, and unless someone who visits points out problems to them they may not notice. It is easy, for example, for an overworked careworker to assume that your relative or friend is just not hungry and to remove an uneaten meal when perhaps s/he actually only needed help in cutting up the food.

The advice above is not supposed to imply that staff in care and nursing homes in general are not kind and caring. However, you will know your own relative or friend best and will be able to spot problems and voice her/his concerns in the most appropriate manner.

Chapter 12

Wills and probate

My father-in-law had made a proper Will and had left a detailed inventory of his property and where documents were to be found. His affairs were in impeccable order and we did not have in this instance to apply for probate. Even so it took my husband, who had been appointed executor, several weeks to sort everything out, and it cost a lot in time, postage and telephone calls. I dread to think of how difficult it must be for someone dealing with a less orderly estate.

****

Many people put off writing a Will because it seems morbid, or because death seems so far away. Many are also under the illusion that if they do not write a Will 'my spouse/children will get everything anyway'. If your relatives, or friends, are under this impression it is important to disabuse them. If someone dies without leaving a Will ('intestate'), then the law has strict criteria about where the money goes and it may not be where your relative, or friend, would choose.

It is very likely that the first time you have to consider this matter is after the death of a relative, perhaps one or other of your parents, and so this section has been written to give some clear guidance to someone dealing with Wills and probate for the first time. Several publications are available which cover the whole subject in more detail and the official probate website is extremely helpful (www.gov.uk/wills-probate-inheritance).

Briefly, if the person you care for has died and left a Will, the procedure is as follows:

1. Read the Will and find out who has been appointed as executor.
2. Inform all the financial institutions involved of the death and of the identity of the executor.
3. Collect details about all bank accounts, stocks and shares, property owned and debts owed to the estate.
4. Collect any details you can find about any debts owed by the person who has died.
5. Apply for probate if necessary.
6. After the grant of probate, collect funds from all bank and financial accounts, pay debts from this sum and pass the rest to the beneficiaries.

If you are helping to sort out the affairs of an elderly relative or friend after the death of her/his spouse, and if the deceased has left a Will, then this is the easiest scenario. However, 'easy' is a relative term. There are many documents which have to be completed, telephone calls which have to be made, and decisions which must be agreed upon. Be prepared for long, frustrating waits on the end of a telephone line, difficult discussions and tedious form completion.

The following tips are intended to be helpful and assist you in avoiding pitfalls. They are not intended to be a complete guide. It is recommended that you borrow or buy a publication which deals with the subject, or download from a website the detailed information for each instance which you might encounter.

Checking the Will

Hopefully the deceased will have written a Will. A Will does not

have to be drawn up by a solicitor, nor does it have to be complicated to be valid. Your relative or friend may have written her/
his own Will, or have used a 'Will form', which can be obtained
from a stationer or a website, or have had a Will drawn up by a
solicitor. You will need to find the Will. Some people lodge their
Will with a bank or a solicitor for safe-keeping; some people just
store it with other important documents in the home. Once you
find the document, keep it safe. It is worth making some photo-
copies to work from and perhaps to distribute to other relatives
if required. The original will be needed if you have to apply for
probate.

A Will should be signed by the person making it and dated,
it should be witnessed by two people who are not beneficiaries, and it should appoint an 'executor'. It is likely that spouses
will appoint each other as executor, in which case the procedure
is fairly simple. Sometimes people appoint more than one
executor. The executor is the person who has the responsibility
for 'administering the estate', which means collecting all the
credit owed and paying all the debts from the estate and then
ensuring that any funds remaining are passed to the beneficiary
or beneficiaries. Some people appoint either a solicitor or a bank
to be executor of their Will, and if this is the case you will need
to contact the executor institution or professional, and they will
continue the procedure as below. If you are the carer of an elderly
relative or friend and that person has been appointed as executor
of a Will, you may have to guide them through the procedures.

Informing those who need to know

Inform all the financial institutions involved of the death and of
the identity of the executor. Any accounts/agreements in joint
names will need to be changed to the name of the surviving account holder. Most organisations are trained to react quickly and
sympathetically to the report of bereavement, and many have

a dedicated bereavement team to deal with changes to account names and any rebates or reductions in payments. (There is more information on this in Chapter 13.)

At the same time as you deal with these financial matters, you could take the opportunity to inform others who need to know. This might include the local library (return library tickets) and relevant social clubs, neighbours and acquaintances, the local hospital if regular outpatients' appointments are kept, the regular caring agency, the hairdresser if appointments are made ahead, and so on. The benefit of trying to inform everyone involved is that it saves difficulty later. It can be really upsetting to a surviving partner or child to receive a reminder from the library about fines due for unreturned books or a friendly call from a fellow churchgoer, for example, and to have to give the news of death all over again.

Do not forget items like satellite TV agreements, broadband or car breakdown agreements. There is often a contract involved with these and the names will have to be changed to keep things valid.

Collect any details you can find about any debts owed by the person who has died. This will include money owing to the Inland Revenue. The Tax Inspector will probably require you to complete a tax return for the portion of the year between the previous April and the death. On receipt of this, the Inland Revenue will inform you if any income tax is owing, or if a rebate is due. You will need all this information for the probate application, if you are making this. In respect of other debts, the executor is responsible for making sure that these have been paid before paying any beneficiaries. There are rules about how to discover debts if you do not know the details. You have to advertise in *The London Gazette* and in a local paper, for anyone who might have a claim on the estate, and wait a certain time before paying any beneficiaries.

If the estate which you are administering is worth more than a certain amount there will be inheritance tax to pay and you will have to calculate this and pay it to the Inland Revenue before probate is granted. You do not always have to go through the process of applying for probate. In certain circumstances you can administer the estate and handle all the affairs of the deceased without probate. These circumstances apply when, for example, the deceased has left very little money or when everything they had was jointly owned with someone to whom the dead person's share passes automatically (for example, between a married couple) and no building society or bank accounts contain large sums of money. You should check with the probate office if this applies in the case you are dealing with. If you are not applying for probate then, as you contact any financial institutions, explain this straightaway. Most institutions have a special form to be completed which enables the account to be transferred into the name of the surviving owner. However, in some cases banks and building societies may insist upon probate being obtained.

****

My sister and I were named as joint executors. On reading the instructions on the probate form, I realised that just one of us could take on the task – the other is allowed to 'opt out' of the administration procedures. However, I was keen for my sister to see that everything was above board and did not suggest this. Later I wished that I had because everything had to be signed by us both. As she lived some distance away this involved a lot of 'to-and-fro' posting of documents and made everything take longer.

****

Applying for probate

The term 'probate' means the issuing of a legal document to one or more people authorising them to administer the estate. The probate registry issues the document, which is called a 'grant of representa-tion'. These are the three types of grant of representation:

1. Probate: Issued to one or more of the executors named in the deceased's Will, where executors have been named and are willing to act.
2. Letters of administration (with Will): Issued when there is a Will, but there is no executor named, or when the executors are unable to apply, or do not wish to be involved in dealing with the estate.
3. Letters of administration: Issued when the deceased had not made a Will, or any Will made is not valid.

If you telephone either the Probate Office or the Inland Revenue and explain the situation, they will normally send you a 'Probate Pack', which contains the probate application form (on which you give details of the deceased and the person applying for grant of probate) and the Account of the Estate form, which asks you to give a full account of the deceased's estate and also a collection of explanatory notes. Don't be put off by the size of the Probate Pack; it contains forms which you may not have to complete, and extensive explanatory notes.

Read through the pack very carefully before you start. Different forms are supplied for different circumstances and it really is easy to begin completing the wrong form and waste a lot of time.

For the Account of the Estate form, you should try to obtain the full value of all items shown. This means that you should try to get estimates and include any interest or bonus that will be paid to bank or building society accounts. You should also ask share companies about dividends which are due. Any money due from the deceased's employer should be included if your relative died whilst still employed, and this may include unpaid salary or a 'death in service' payment. The full market value of any house should be shown, although a professional valuation is not normally required. You can give an informed estimate simply by checking with a local estate agent. The value of household goods, jewellery and belongings should be shown as the amount for which they could be sold, and you are generally allowed to make an estimate of this. This form looks extremely complicated, but you will probably find that you only have to complete a few parts of it. The explanatory notes are very helpful, and usually included in the Probate Pack is a flow chart which helps you to work out what to do at each stage of the procedure. The Probate Office helpline is also very helpful, and telephone queries are answered promptly.

****

The Probate form asked some very detailed questions about my father-in-law's brothers, sisters, parents and even aunts and uncles! We really didn't know the answers and the explanatory notes didn't help on this question. But when we telephoned the Probate Office, they told us that we could just put 'unknown' and the problem was solved. Apparently they would be more likely to need this information if the deceased had died intestate.

****

As well as ensuring that you collect proper details of the worth of the estate, make sure that you keep all details and receipts of any expenses incurred. Certain expenses are allowed to be offset against the estate before inheritance tax is calculated, and you should be sure to do this if you wish to minimise the inheritance tax bill. Some of these allowable expenses are clear, such as the funeral director's bill, and others are more vague. For example, you can claim miscellaneous 'mourning expenses', which might include the cost of getting to the funeral venue or of purchasing suitable clothing to wear to the funeral. You can claim for the cost of a headstone, and for the costs of the refreshments after the funeral.

If you are reading this section in order to deal with the estate of someone who has already died, it may be too late to do more than the above in order to minimise inheritance tax, but if you are guiding your elderly relative or friend through making a Will, then it is wise to get proper advice about legal ways to avoid inheritance tax. Many financial institutions and firms of solicitors specialise in this area and a consultation with one of these will be well worth the cost involved.

It may take several weeks, or even months, to get all the information together and submit the forms. The forms are submitted to the Probate Office where you wish to go for interview. Most people think they have to go to the office nearest the deceased's home, but you can choose the office most convenient for you (and any other executors) to attend. The Probate Office will send you a date and time for the interview. The interview is very brief and simply consists of a formal oath that what you have declared is the truth. You can take someone with you to the Probate Office if you wish, but normally you will be interviewed alone.

After the Grant of Probate

After the interview the Grant of Probate will be sent to you within a very few days and you can then notify all the financial institutions (and anyone else) and proceed to pay bills and share out the estate.

****

There was a final share dividend payment which we had to claim and the institution made out a cheque in the names of both my brothers and myself as we were all executors. This made life very difficult as we did not have a joint account and could not pay it into any of our bank accounts. We had to write and ask for the cheque to be made out to just my elder brother (he then shared the money out) but we all had to sign the letter and it caused quite a delay. The bank later told us that we could have opened a joint account for the purposes of administration of the estate.

****

If there is inheritance tax to pay, probate will not be granted until it has been paid. This can appear to be a 'catch 22' situation. If probate has not been granted, how can you obtain the money to pay the inheritance tax? Fortunately many banks and building societies will release money for this purpose from the deceased's account. But they don't always tell you this until you ask!

****

I was amazed to find out how expensive the funeral costs were. My father had asked for the simplest possible coffin and funeral arrangements, but there were some problems. Firstly, other members of the family wanted different arrangements (a better coffin was one demand). I also found that even a 'simple' funeral was not cheap. Fortunately the Funeral Directors explained to me that the bank would release the money from Dad's account to pay for the funeral. I don't think we could have afforded it otherwise.

****

After probate has been granted it is up to the executor to pay any other debts on the estate. If there is not enough money to pay all the debts, there is a certain order in which they have to be paid. This order is as follows: first any funeral expenses and expenses involved in dealing with the Will, then the Inland Revenue & Customs, any social security debts and any unpaid pension or wages contributions.

Living Wills

'Living Wills' are not really Wills as such. They are more accurately described as Advance Directives on stopping life-prolonging treatment. Making an Advance Directive does not obviate the need to make a proper Will, which will come into force upon the death of the person making it. With the advance of medical science there is ever greater potential for individuals to be 'kept alive' without any real prospect of their being able to live independently at any time in the future. An Advance Directive allows you to state under what conditions you would like to refuse life-sustaining treatment.

Although doctors and other medical professionals may take your views stated in any Advance Statement* into account, they are not legally bound to do so if they believe that acting on your views is not in your best interests medically. An Advance Directive has a different standing (it is legally binding in England and Wales), and your doctors should follow your instructions.

If the person you care for would like to make an Advance Directive, there are a few simple rules that should be followed:

- The document needs to be clear and concise
- It is helpful if it considers the types of treatment that the person concerned would not like to undergo and gives reasons. (This will help others to assess whether they would have consented to a specific treatment)
- It is worth getting the document witnessed by two people, who, preferably, will not benefit after the death
- It is also worth consulting the GP.

You can store a 'Living Will' with an original (after death) Will but make sure that it can be accessed easily. Most importantly, your relative or friend needs to make sure that someone (the next of kin) knows of its existence, otherwise it may not be acted upon. If you have granted Lasting Power of Attorney (health and welfare) to someone else, then you need to ensure that s/he is conversant with the terms of any Advance Directive as the two may conflict with each other.

---

*An 'Advance Statement' allows you to make your views known, in advance, about your preferences for medical and other treatment. It differs from an Advance Directive in being merely a statement of your views and is not legally binding on medical professionals.

Chapter 13

After a bereavement

My mother had become more and more frail in the two years before my father died. To be honest we all thought that she would be the first to go. Then my father died very suddenly after a short illness and we realised the extent of Mother's need for help in many areas of her life. I also realised that I had become her chief carer. What took me aback was how many small everyday things I had to sort out so soon after his death – even things like re-arranging the electricity and gas bills. She just wasn't up to it.

****

Service utilities and financial issues

This chapter focuses on what needs to be done when an elderly person loses her/his partner, generally through bereavement, though much of the information below is also relevant if the partner has to move into institutional care and can no longer remain with her/him at home.

When someone dies there are many things that have to be tackled immediately after and in connection with the death – things like registration of the death, administering the Will and arranging the funeral. But there may also be multiple small practical considerations which need to be addressed simply to enable the surviving member of a partnership to continue her/

his everyday life. It often falls to the carer to deal with these issues. There are likely to be many changes needed to documentation, and some practical changes as well to help the surviving partner manage alone.

Changes to documentation

Any accounts/agreements in joint names will need to be changed to the name of the surviving account holder. There may be many more of these than are at first apparent. One way to find out is to go back through the bank statements and note all automatic payments out. This should reveal most commitments, such as council tax, rental agreements, insurances and membership fees. Remember that some direct debits and standing orders are only paid annually so check at least a year's worth of statements.

A simple method is to write two lists, one for those items where the account name needs to be changed and one for items needing cancellation. Most organisations will accept simple changes of name via the telephone, but unless you hold Power of Attorney most will want to speak to the remaining account holder rather than a third party. If the person you care for is unable to make the whole call, most organisations will accept her/his verification of name and account details and verbal permission to allow you to do the rest.

The good news is that most organisations are trained to react quickly and sympathetically to the report of a bereavement, and many have a dedicated bereavement team to deal with changes to account names and any rebates or reductions in payments. The not-so-good news is that many organisations have call centres to which any call is automatically routed, and call centre staff are trained to respond in an automatic way. A good tip is to avoid answering any routine security questions and state immediately that you wish to report a death.

Don't allow this:

'Hello, this is General Bank Plc, Robin speaking. Can I have your sort code please?'

'Er, yes – it's 61-75-94.'

'And your account number please.'

'52305769.'

'Account in the name of Charles and Vera Johnson. Can you give me your pass code please?'

'Er, no, I haven't got that, I...'

'I'm afraid I'll have to ask you some security questions then. What is your mother's maiden name?'

Instead:

'Hello, this is General Bank Plc, Robin speaking. Can I have your sort code please?'

'Good morning. My name is Valerie Johnson and I wish to record the death of my father-in-law, Charles Johnson. Would you put me through to the correct department please.'

'Certainly. One moment please.'

Many organisations will require a copy of the death certificate (not a photocopy). When registering a death it is worth getting several copies of the death certificate at the time. The registrar will give you as many as you need, but there is a small payment for each one. However, the payment is higher if you have to ask for extra copies later.

State pensions and council tax

When a death is registered the Registrar will normally ask for details of any pensions that are being administered by the state or by any public organisation such as the Armed Forces or the Civil Service. If possible, remember to take details of these pensions with you when you register the death. The Registrar will then inform the pension administrators of the death. Within a short time (days rather than weeks) the pension organisation will contact the widow or widower to follow up. If there is a widow's pension payable there will probably be some forms to complete but because the notification has come via the Registrar you may not need to forward a death certificate.

Many Registrars will also inform the local council of the death. One person living alone is eligible for a lower rate of council tax and a rebate of any overpayment previously made. Most councils will arrange this immediately they are informed of the death but if the widow or widower does not receive notification within a few weeks the matter should be followed up with the council concerned. If council tax is being paid by direct debit any rebate or adjustment will be made directly into the bank account from which the payment is made. Again you are unlikely to be asked for the death certificate in this case. Remember to check bank statements after the due date of the next payment to make sure your instructions have been acted upon.

Insurances

All insurance companies have dedicated bereavement teams who normally deal with any claims or administrative changes quickly. Life insurance companies will require an original copy of the death certificate but many property insurance companies do not, and will change the account details if you telephone them to explain. Be careful to ensure that you notify the company of all policies held and do not rely on their systems to work in your favour.

****

I notified the insurance company of my mother's death and they dealt with the notification and the claim quickly and efficiently. However, a couple of months later, when I was going through some of my mother's papers, I discovered a second 'live' policy with the same company. Although they dealt with the second claim just as competently, I felt that this smacked of 'sharp practice'. I am sure their computer systems must have shown that there was more than one policy in my mother's name and that they deliberately avoided telling me about it.

****

Car insurance may have to be completely re-assessed and a new policy issued depending upon whether the deceased or the remaining partner was the main insured driver.

Banks and building societies

Financial organisations generally have robust procedures for dealing with bereavement. They will need to see an original copy of the death certificate. It may be useful to go into the branch of the organisation concerned rather than try to write or telephone. The clerk at the branch will then photocopy the death certificate, certify it as a true copy and return it to you. You can also usually complete any forms required on the spot. A joint account can usually be altered to continue in one name only, with the minimum of trouble. However, it may be the case that only one partner (often the man) held the account in his name and dealt with all the finances. If this is the case, a new bank or building society account will need to be set up and each bank has its own regulations concerning this. You will need to enquire about these. At this stage, consider whether to set up a joint account with the person you care for, or whether to organise a Lasting Power of Attorney (see Chapter 2 on Financial matters). It may save you a lot of trouble later if you think about this now. Any debit cards on the account will probably need to be re-issued. If the bank forgets to mention this, make sure that you ask them about it.

Credit cards

Credit card companies also have standard procedures for dealing with bereavement. Cards held in the sole name of the remaining partner will not be affected. However, where the remaining partner was only a secondary cardholder with a credit card company, the account is not automatically changed to their name. The company will cancel the card and the remaining partner will have to re-apply in her/his own right for a card if this is required. Nor as a general rule do card companies transfer a balance from the card of the deceased partner to the remaining partner. Any balances on credit cards are considered to be a debt on the estate and are due for payment, though interest is frozen on death. However, some credit card companies adopt a compassionate approach and actually cancel a debt on the death of the cardholder. You will need to ascertain the exact position with the individual company.

Rental agreements and utility bills

Ongoing rental agreements for items such as satellite television and telephones can usually be switched to the name of the remaining partner. Often the companies do not even require a copy of the death certificate, and will make the switch once you confirm the details over the telephone, provided the payments continue to be made from the same bank account as before. The same applies to utility bills. Items no longer required (for example, car breakdown insurance if the remaining partner does not drive and intends to sell the car) may need to be cancelled in writing. If such an agreement is annually renewed, a rebate for the unused portion of the agreement should be issued to the estate. If the remaining partner is now in a straitened financial situation this would be the right time to investigate help with paying for utilities. There are national, local and charitable grants available to help people with low incomes in these circumstances.

Practical matters concerning everyday living

Even if completely physically fit and mentally capable, the person you are caring for may have problems dealing with some everyday tasks. Elderly people have often over the years developed their partnership so that only one of them carries out certain tasks. It is not uncommon, for example, to find that elderly men have no notion of cookery. Similarly, the elderly women of today were born into a generation where it was common for only the man to be the car driver or to manage the finances.

****

My father always operated the DVD player and when he died my mother had no idea how to work it. She was also partially sighted, which meant that she had difficulty in reading the instruction book or seeing the control buttons. Eventually we bought her a DVD player which was much simpler to operate, and because the instructions appeared on the screen she was able to see them and to learn to operate it after a fashion.

****

It may be up to you as the carer to assess the gaps in capabilities, and of course it may require tact and diplomacy both to discover and to address these gaps. Lack of practical skills can be overcome in a number of ways. If your elderly relative or friend is amenable to learning a new skill this helps, but sometimes you may encounter resistance. On the other hand, many elderly people actually seem to gain a new lease of life after overcoming the initial shock of the death of a partner. They discover untapped depths within themselves. In this case there are many resources open to them. Local authorities offer (for example) classes in simple cookery, car maintenance, or basic house maintenance, and most of these classes positively welcome older people. Senior citizens usually receive a discount on the price of classes and, as an added extra, may make new acquaintances whilst attending them. You can research such classes either on the web or via your local library. The library and the internet are in nearly all cases invaluable sources of local information.

Sometimes the person you care for may not want to learn a skill but may be quite amenable to making changes to get around the lack of it. For example, an elderly person may not want or be able to learn to cook. There are several alternatives to them cooking for themselves. Or they may not want to be bothered or may be unable to learn the ins and outs of how bank accounts and bill-paying work. There are ways of helping with this.

Meals and cooking

Meals-on-wheels

The meals-on-wheels (it may have another name depending on the area) scheme is operated by the local authority (LA) and you will need to contact them to find out what (if anything) is available. Most LAs specify that the service is only available to those who are unable to cook a meal themselves, but each has its own criteria to decide this. The person you are caring for will possibly have to be assessed by social services against the LA criteria. Some LAs will not supply meals if there is a carer available to do so. Some will offer cooked meals only; others will supply cook-chill meals, which can be reheated or microwaved; some will offer a choice or a mixture of both. Mostly these meals are delivered only once a day in the middle of the day and other arrangements will have to be made for breakfast and evening meals. The meals-on-wheels service is not free and will have to be paid for. It is normally a flat-rate charge, usually below the cost of buying a hot meal elsewhere.

Ready meals

For someone who is able to operate a cooker or a microwave but who does not want to be bothered with cooking from scratch, there are a whole range of frozen and cook-chill meals available in every supermarket. The meals range from simple 'boil in the bag' items such as rice or microwaveable bags of fresh vegetables to complete 'roast dinners'. Most of them are very appetising and nutritionally adequate. Your relative or friend will probably need a freezer to use this option unless shopping can be arranged several times each week. There are also a number of firms who will deliver these frozen or cook-chill meals, which can be chosen in advance from a range of menus.

Caring agencies

Most agency carers are happy to prepare a meal and serve it up, but the amount of preparation time for a meal produced from fresh ingredients may make this an expensive option as agencies usually operate hourly charges (see Chapter 9 on Professional carers).

Neighbours and friends

Friends or neighbours who are at home during the day may be prepared to cook an extra portion when they cook for themselves and to carry it round to your relative or friend. This may not be a perfect answer because you would have to be sure that the neighbour or friend would be prepared to do this on a regular basis. You would also have to be prepared to make other arrangements to cover times when this person was on holiday or out for the day. However, it is certainly a solution worth investigating, especially as a stop-gap.

Financial solutions

Joint accounts

If the person you care for is happy to trust you in financial matters, and you are happy to help in this area, a good solution is to set up a joint bank account so that you can deal with bills, check that deposits from pensions etc are being made and keep an eye on things generally. The bank branch where her/his account is held will be able to help with this.

Power of Attorney

You and the person you care for may wish to consider Power of Attorney as an option. If the person you care for sets up a Power of Attorney naming you as the attorney you will then have the power to manage all her/his financial affairs for her/him. There are many factors to consider and it may be worth consulting a solicitor, but you can get information from The Public Guardianship Office. One thing you must be aware of is that only Lasting Power of Attorney allows someone to appoint an attorney to handle welfare decisions as well as financial ones. An Enduring Power of Attorney, whilst still perfectly valid, only covers financial affairs (see page 22).

Direct debits

Many utilities and rental firms will happily organise direct debit or standing order payments for their services, and this may work very well. Bills are sent out as before but the amount required to pay the bill is collected via a direct debit. This needs to be set up with each individual utility or rental company, but is a very good way of ensuring regular payment, especially if, as sometimes happens, the person you care for 'forgets' or 'loses' mail.

****

My mother-in-law couldn't cope with the bill paying etc, but wanted to feel that she was in control. We set up direct debit payments for electricity, gas and telephone and this meant that there were never any 'red' bills but at the same time she felt that she knew what was going on.

****

Gardening and house maintenance

If the person you care for is unable to cope with simple things like mowing the lawn or changing lightbulbs, it probably means that either you, as the carer, or friends and neighbours will have to help out. For more complicated tasks such as hedge cutting, plumbing and electrical problems you may need to call on outside help, and this will usually have to be paid for. Indeed, paying for regular help in the garden or for large but irregular tasks such as decorating the house is a good solution provided your relative or friend can afford this. However (and particularly if the financial situation is difficult), there are alternatives.

Social services and local authorities: Social services do not usually provide this type of help but they may have information as to what is available locally, and if the person you are caring for qualifies for financial assistance, then social services may help to organise the care. Local authorities may run schemes to help with house maintenance or house alterations to make life easier for frail elderly people. Enquire at the local library, the Citizens Advice Bureau or check the Local Authority website.

Local charities: Local schemes are often in place to help elderly or disabled people. The local Lions club, Rotaract (the 'action' branch of the Rotary Club) and local Scout Groups are likely sources of help. It is not always easy to find information about what help these groups might offer but the best starting point to find a contact for such groups is your local library.

Churches and clubs: If the person you care for is or was a regular churchgoer, approach the church concerned via the priest or minister. Even where there is no regular helping scheme in place, for such things church congregations will often rally to help someone in need. Similarly, if your relative or friend was a regular member of a local social club it may be worth approaching its members to ask for help. There may be a keen gardener or DIY expert who will be happy to help.

Making changes: Some elderly people may just be resistant to new or different things. They are capable of independent thought and action but just seem to be stubborn and unable to change. In such cases you sometimes have to insist. They may understand 'I want to help but I really can't manage every day', or 'We are not well ourselves and cannot do these things', or 'Let me help you set this up and then you will have control', but equally they may not. For your own sanity you may just have to overrule them. It isn't the best way but it may be the only way. Certainly, if you can arrange that the whole family is in agreement on any approach to change it will make implementing necessary alterations much easier. Family, or group, meetings and agreement are vital at this point.

****

My mother-in-law would not accept any help in the house. Then my husband suffered a stroke. I simply said, 'You are having this outside help because your son is ill and he and I cannot cope at this moment without this extra help.' She accepted it very grudgingly as an interim thing but the door had been opened and everything was easier afterwards.

****

General health

This is a good time to ensure co-ordination of health provision. The person you care for may see the family GP regularly, and possibly the district nursing service will have been in contact. But if s/he and her/his former partner were in generally good health they may not have seen their doctor for months or even years.

GPs in the NHS may have up to 3000 patients on their list and it is very easy to slip through any safety net there is. Some people have a particular dislike of visiting the doctor and may put up with all sorts of discomfort to avoid this. In such a case there may be a build-up of multiple health problems, some of which may only become apparent when the elderly person loses the regular support s/he received from a partner. For example, someone whose eyesight has been failing may have managed adequately and even kept her/his poor sight a secret whilst the partner was around to help out but when forced to live alone problems arise.

Poor sight, bad teeth, neglected feet and deafness are health problems which are all worth tackling, as sometimes small adjustments, like a stronger pair of spectacles or treatment from a chiropodist, may be of immense help and enable the person you care for to live a more independent, better-quality life.

If the person you care for has any of these minor health problems check out the facilities in the area where s/he lives. The first point of information is the GP surgery and the district nursing service (sometimes called the community nursing service). Be persistent. Some GPs may be vague about what is available and unfortunately too aware of their budget restrictions. Some are uninterested in the elderly and their problems. Generally, the district nursing team are likely to be very helpful and will be able to point you in the right direction.

Major changes are taking place in the area of district/community nursing, particularly with regard to elderly care, and there is a big push to improve 'care in the community' to ensure that more elderly people are able to continue living at home and avoid undue hospitalisation. Like many NHS initiatives, it is a money-saving exercise, but there are many benefits to the elderly person wishing to live independently at home. As with other services, the availability and variety of facilities offered differs from area to area (for example, the person in charge may be called a 'community matron' or a 'team leader' depending on the area) but the district nursing team will be able to tell you what is available for your relative or friend. There are also often helpful leaflets or notices in the GP surgery that can tell you what is available.

****

We bought a raised toilet seat and frame for my mother-in-law and fitted grab rails in the bathroom at our own expense. She found them useful but it was only a few months later when we had to call in the district nurse on a health matter that she told us that a proper occupational therapy assessment would have recommended exactly the right height seat and frame for my mother-in-law and that we might have been able to obtain these aids free of charge. We didn't know this level of service was available.

****

Problems with vision: For some visual problems, a sight test and a new prescription for spectacles are all that is needed. It is not generally known that optometry (sight tests) can be done in the home for those who are unable to leave the house. However, the facilities are usually better at the optometrist's practice. If you speak to the receptionist at your relative or friend's local optometry practice beforehand, they will very often make special provision for an elderly person with exceptional difficulties. For example, you might ask if you can use the staff car park if the person you care for cannot walk far. All optometry centres will be able to provide information about free eye tests, and help with provision of spectacles for those unable to pay. If the person you care for is partially sighted, many aids are available for everyday living (see Chapter 1 on First steps). In addition, it is worth contacting the various associations for the blind to see what they can offer (see page 212 for RNIB contact details).

Chapter 13

My elderly aunt was told during an eye examination that the optician had noticed some changes and that he would refer her to her GP as she might need treatment for diabetes. She didn't understand at all. It was only after we asked questions on her behalf that we realised that the eye examination can show up many incipient medical problems (for example, diabetes).

Hearing: Hearing tests are available at home in the same way as sight tests, but again the equipment is better at the hearing centre. The district nursing team will be able to tell you what is available, but the person you care for may need to be referred by the GP. Many private companies offer hearing tests and hearing aids, and some of these are an improvement on what is available on the NHS, but be aware that they will have an interest in providing the latest and most sophisticated alternatives. It may be that your friend or relative needs something much simpler that is easy for them to operate. (Be warned: if you send to hearing aid companies for any catalogues you may remain on their mailing lists for life!)

Chiropody: Again, this is supposed to be available to those who are elderly and/or housebound and who also have an additional health problem requiring visiting 'domiciliary' services. This means that the chiropodist will come out to treat your relative or friend at home. Ask the district nursing team what is available in your area. If you are prepared to pay for the service, it is usually easy to get a chiropodist to do a home visit. If the person you care for attends a day care centre, this service is often offered there.

In conclusion

It may need some pressure on your part to get the services described in this chapter and unfortunately those who make the most fuss are the most likely to get the most complete help. Do not be put off by stories of understaffing or long waits for treatment. Your relative or friend has the right to these services. If s/he has to wait this is still better than getting no help at all. Again, persistence pays off. If you know s/he has been placed on a waiting list, check regularly to see what the position is.

For the more active elderly, treatment for minor problems, dental work, occupational therapy and physiotherapy, and even some out-patient services, may be supplied at local 'community' hospitals which are more accessible and pleasant to visit than large general hospitals. Many areas offer a transport service (staffed by volunteers) to get people who are not car drivers to doctors, out-patient appointments and therapeutic services. The GP surgery should have details of this service if you ask (see Chapter 3 on Getting about).

If the person you care for has the means and can pay for private treatment, the whole process may be quicker and simpler. Again, the GP surgery may carry lists of local practitioners of chiropody and physiotherapy, and they will probably be prepared to come to the home if necessary, but it will be expensive. If you need to find practitioners yourself, local libraries, telephone books and, increasingly, the internet are good sources of information.

Appendix

Further useful information

Chapter 1: First steps

Disabled Living Foundation
Provides information and
advice on equipment. There is
an Equipment Demonstration
Centre with large displays of
equipment which visitors can
try out and where advice can
be obtained.
Helpline: 0845 130 9177
(charged at local call rate)
Equipment Demonstration
Centre: (020) 7289 6111 ext 247
www.dlf.org.uk

**Assist-UK Disabled Living
Centres**
A network of centres around
the UK which provide
information and advice on
products and where you
can see and try out products.
Tel: 0161 832 9757
www.assist-uk.org

British Red Cross
Ability Catalogue – products for
independence.
Tel: 0844 893 0090
www.redcross.org.uk

Incontinence Products
Tel: 0800 180 4325
www.dryforlife.co.uk

Lloyds Pharmacy
Local pharmacy branches
stock catalogues of aids and
equipment and can order items
for you and have them delivered
to your nearest pharmacy. The
website has a 'nearest pharmacy'
search facility.
www.lloydspharmacy.co.uk

Independent Living
Provides impartial information
for family carers, care professionals and individuals with a
disability, about products and

services to help with mobility and independence.
www.independentliving.co.uk

Benefitsnow online shop
For elastic shoe laces and other aids for living.
Tel: 0845 459 6006
www.co-opmobility.co.uk

Gimble – hands-free reading device
Tel: 01743 289288
www.gimbleuk.com

Independent Occupational Therapy
Occupational therapists in independent practice.
Tel: 0800 389 4873
www.cotss-ip.org.uk

Royal National Institute for the Blind (RNIB)
Tel: 0303 123 9999
www.rnib.org.uk

Action on Hearing Loss
Online shop with aids for everyday living for the deaf.
Tel: 0808 808 0123
Textphone: 0808 808 9000
www.actiononhearingloss.org.uk

Telecare
Tel: 0300 123 1002 (free leaflet)
www.nhs.uk/Planners/Yourhealth/Pages/Telecare.aspx

Chapter 2: Financial matters

Citizens Advice Bureau
The Citizens Advice service helps people resolve their legal, financial and other problems by providing free, independent and confidential advice.
Local telephone numbers can be found on their website or via directory inquiries.
www.citizensadvice.org.uk

Government services
Information about government services, tax, benefits and pensions and other government regulated financial matters such as power of attorney can now all be found on one central website.
www.gov.uk

Department of Work and Pensions
www.dwp.gov.uk

Co-operative Mobility
This site enables you to assess yourself for Disability Living Allowance or Attendance Allowance before you apply. You can find out whether you qualify and at what rate you are likely to be paid.
Tel: 0845 459 6006
www.co-opmobility.co.uk

Independent Age
Aims to provides lifelong support for the elderly on very low incomes.
Tel: 0845 262 1863
www.independentage.org

Nursing Home Fees Agency
Gives advice on funding Nursing Home Fees.
Tel: 01865 733000
www.nhfa.co.uk

Chapter 3: Getting about

Department for Transport
General information about transport facilities for the elderly.
www.dft.gov.uk

Blue Badge scheme
www.direct.gov.uk/DisabledPeople

Disability Rights UK (RADAR)
Tel: 020 7250 3222
www.radar-shop.org.uk

Stairlifts

Stannah
Tel: 0800 715171
www.stannah.com

Brooks stairlifts
Tel: 0800 834730
www.brooksstairlifts.co.uk

Walking aids

Uniscan Walkers
Tel: 0800 064 0762
www.uniscan-walkers.co.uk

Able Mail Order
Tel: 0800 358 0445
www.independentliving.co.uk/product1.html

Plus organisations listed under 'Chapter 1: First steps'

Chapter 4: Nutrition

Learning to Cook by Marion Cunningham.
Publisher: Knopf, 1999.

How to Boil an Egg: ... And 184 Other Simple Recipes for One by Jan Arkless.
Publisher: Elliott Right Way Books, 1997.

Wiltshire Farm Foods

Deliver frozen ready meals to your home.
Tel: 0800 773773
www.wiltshirefarmfoods.com

Women's Royal Voluntary Service (WRVS)

Deliver ready meals to your home.
Tel: 0845 600 5885
www.wrvs.org.uk/how-we-help/practical-support-at-home/meals-on-wheels

Oakhouse Foods

Deliver frozen ready-meals to your home.
Tel: 0845 643 2009
www.oakhousefoods.co.uk/meals-desserts-2

British Dental Association

To search for a dentist who specialises in elderly or reluctant patients.
www.bda-dentistry.org.uk

Chapter 5: Social needs

Contact the Elderly

Sunday afternoon tea for lonely people (restricted areas).
Tel: 0800 716543
www.contact-the-elderly.org.uk

Cruse Bereavement Care

Help, counselling and support for the bereaved.
Helpline: 0844 477 9400
www.crusebereavementcare.org.uk

Royal National Institute for the Blind (RNIB)

Talking books and other products for the blind and partially sighted.
Tel: 0303 123 9999
www.rnib.org.uk

Action on Hearing Loss

Online shop with aids for everyday living for the deaf.
Tel: 0808 808 0123

Textphone: 0808 808 9000
www.actiononhearingloss.org.uk

Windsor Products
Books like *Master your computer*
and freebies for older folk.
Tel: 0871 224 0777
www.windsorproducts.com

Gardening for Disabled Trust
The Trust gives grants to
people all over the United
Kingdom in order that they
may continue to garden,
despite advancing illness, age
or disability.
Contact: The Secretary,
Gardening for Disabled Trust,
Hayes Farmhouse, Hayes
Lane,
Peasmarsh, Rye, East Sussex
TN31 6XR

Chapter 6: Recognising medical conditions

The Stroke Association
Tel: 020 7566 0300
www.stroke.org.uk

British Heart Foundation
Tel: 0300 330 3322
www.bhf.org.uk

Diabetes UK
Tel: 020 7424 1000
www.diabetes.org.uk

For dementia, see Chapter 7
below.

Chapter 7: Dealing with dementia

The Alzheimer's Society
UK's leading care and research
charity for people with
dementia, their families and
carers.
Tel: 0300 222 1122 (national
helpline)
www.alzheimers.org.uk

Alzheimer Scotland
Tel: 0808 808 3000 (helpline)
www.alzscot.org

Dementia UK
Seeks to improve the quality of
life for people affected
by dementia.
Helpline: 0845 257 9406
www.dementiauk.org

Dementia Ireland
Tel: +353 (0)1 416 2035
www.dementia.ie

Chapter 8: Caring for the carer

Independent Age

Information for the elderly and for carers. Also provides lifelong support for the elderly on very low incomes.
Tel: 0845 262 1863
www.independentage.org

Carers UK

(Links to sites for Scotland, Wales and Northern Ireland).
Tel: 020 7378 4999
www.carersuk.org

Carers Trust

Tel: (London office) 0844 800 4361
Tel: (Glasgow office) 0141 221 5066
www.carers.org

Civil Service Retirement Fellowship

The Civil Service Retirement Fellowship exists to help retired civil servants (home visits, local newsletters and group social events). Both retired and serving civil servants can join the Fellowship.
Tel: 020 8691 7411
www.csrf.org.uk

Soldiers, Sailors, Airmen and Families Association (SSAFA)

National charity helping serving and ex-service men, women and their families, including widows and widowers in need.
Tel: 020 7403 8783
www.ssafa.org.uk

The Royal British Legion

Provides financial, social and emotional support to those who have served and are currently serving in the Armed Forces, and their dependants.
Tel: 020 3207 2100
www.britishlegion.org.uk

Co-operative Mobility

This site enables you to assess yourself for Disability Living Allowance or Attendance Allowance before you apply. You can find out whether you qualify and at what rate you are likely to be paid.
Tel: 0845 459 6006
www.co-opmobility.co.uk

End of Life, the Essential Guide to Caring by Mary Jordan and Judy Carole Kauffmann. Publisher: Hammersmith

Health Books
www.endoflifebook.com

Chapter 9: Care agencies and professional carers

UK Home Care Association
Tel: 020 8288 1551
www.ukhca.co.uk

Find Me Good Care
Set up by the Social Care
Institute for Excellence.
www.findmegoodcare.co.uk

SUPRA UK
Outdoor keysafes to hold the
door key to your relative or
friend's house securely.
Tel: 08700 539723
www.keysafe.co.uk

Services provided by your local
authority will be listed in your
local library and on the individual local authority websites.

Useful sources of information
about care fees include:

Age UK
www.ageuk.org.uk/home-
and-care/care-homes/

PayingforCare
Lists specialist financial
advisors in different areas.
www.payingforcare.org

Chapter 10: Managing change

Cruse Bereavement Care
Help, counselling and support
for the bereaved.
Helpline: 0844 477 9400
www.crusebereavementcare.
org.uk

Disabled Living Foundation
Provides information and
advice on equipment. There is
an equipment demonstration
centre with large displays of
items which visitors can try
out and where advice can be
obtained.
Helpline: 0845 130 9177
(charged at local call rate)
Equipment Demonstration
Centre: (020) 7289 6111 ext 247
www.dlf.org.uk

Assist-UK Disabled Living Centres
A network of centres around
the UK, which provide
information and advice on

products and where you
can see and try these out.
Tel: 0161 832 9757
www.assist-uk.org

Chapter 11: Choosing a care home or nursing home

Age UK
www.ageuk.org.uk/home-
and-care/care-homes/

The Elderly Accommodation Counsel
For lists of homes in most areas.
Tel: 0800 377 7070
www.eac.org.uk

The Registered Nursing Home Association
For a list of registered nursing homes.
Tel: 0800 074 0194 (Freephone)
www.rnha.co.uk

The Money Advice Service
Offers information about
funding long-term care
Tel: 0300 500 5000 (English)
Tel: 0300 500 5555 (Welsh)
www.moneyadviceservice.org.uk

Alzheimers Society
Factsheet available: *Paying for care.*
www.alzheimers.org.uk

Nursing Home Fees Agency
Gives advice on funding
nursing home fees.
Tel: 01865 733000
www.nhfa.co.uk

Chapter 12: Wills and probate

HM Court Service
For advice about Wills and probate.
Tel: 020 7189 2000
www.justice.gov.uk/about/hmcts

HM Revenue and Customs
For specific advice about
probate and inheritance tax.
Tel: 0845 302 0900
www.hmrc.gov.uk/inheritancetax

Community Legal Service
Free leaflets on Wills and probate.
Tel: 0845 345 4345
www.clsdirect.org.uk

Age UK
Fact sheet on Living Wills.
Tel: 0800 169 6565
www.ageuk.org.uk/

money-matters/legal-issues/
living-wills

Chapter 13: After a bereavement

British Association of Occupational Therapists
Tel: 020 7357 6480
www.cot.co.uk

The Outside Clinic
Offers eye tests and an eyecare service in your own home.
Tel: 0800 85 4477
www.outsideclinic.com

Wiltshire Farm Foods
Delivers frozen ready-meals to your home
Tel: 0800 773773
www.wiltshirefarmfoods.com

Women's Royal Voluntary Service (WRVS)
Meals-on-wheels and social transport schemes; a good-neighbour scheme for minor household repairs.
www.wrvs.org.uk
0845 600 5885

Foundations
Information on local home improvement agencies to help older people stay in their own homes.
Tel: 0845 864 5210
www.foundations.uk.com

Office of the Public Guardian
Information about Power of Attorney.
Tel: 0300 456 0300
www.justice.gov.uk/about/opg

Rotaract
The 'active' branch of Rotary Clubs for younger members; organises activities such as gardening and helping the elderly.
Tel: local telephone numbers
www.rotaract.org.uk

Lions Clubs International
Local volunteer helpers.
Tel: 0121 441 4544
www.lions105m.org.uk

The Scout Movement
Local groups may be prepared to give active help to individual elderly people. To find your local groups contact the national HQ.
Tel: 0845 300 1818
www.scouts.org.uk

Index

Civil Service Retirement
  Fellowship, 216
cleaning and other household
  duties, 6–8, 205–206
  help with, 140–141, 161–163,
  205–206
  see also washing oneself
clothes (and getting dressed/
  undressed), 9–10, 163, 167
  dementia and, 111–112
clubs and organisations, local
  (cared-for's), 129, 205–206
Code of Practice (Mental
  Capacity Act), 121
Cold Weather Payments, 31
commercial sources *see* private
  and commercial sources
communal (common) area in
  residential home, 171,
  177–178
community', 'care in the, 5,
  127, 207
community or district nurse,
  4, 14, 46, 93, 133, 151, 154,
  158, 171, 206, 207–208
community hospital, 4, 78,
  103, 210
Community Legal Service, 218
companionship, agencies
  providing, 141–142
computers, 69, 70, 77, 160
  online/internet entertainment,
  31, 69, 75, 176
concussion, 92
confabulation, 54, 115, 151
Constant Attendance
  Allowance, 30
Contact the Elderly, 214
conversation problems, 84,
  115–119
cooker, 7, 121, 159, 202
  microwave, 7, 57, 64, 159,
  160, 202, 203
cooking, 52, 55, 57, 74–75, 124,
  202–203
  learning, 54, 74, 216
  in nursing homes, 180
Co-Operative Mobility,
  213, 216

council tax, 31, 197–198
crafts, 72–73
Cruse Bereavement Care, 214,
  217
cupboards, dry-food storage,
  56

daily living, 71–72
  bereaved persons, 201–209
  in residential homes, 180–182
day (and date)
  care agency availability, 143–144
  forgetting/unawareness, 83,
  107, 108
  see also time
day centres, 42, 58, 75, 78–79,
  112
deafness *see* hearing problems
death
  certification, 197, 198, 199,
  200
  documentation changes, 196–197
  informing those who need
  to know, 187–189
  see also bereavement;
  probate; Wills
debit cards, 25, 135, 199
debt, 186, 187, 188, 193, 200
delusions in dementia, 84
dementia, 81–86, 105–121
  alarm call systems and, 97
  anti-social feelings/
  behaviour, 79
  care homes for those with,
  168, 182
  day centres, 78
  driving and, 39
  hospital admission (for
  accident), 101
  nutrition and food issues,
  53–54, 57
  support organisations,
  215
  vascular, 81, 82, 105, 128
Dementia Ireland, 215
Dementia UK, 215
dentist, 214
  see also teeth
denture problems, 52, 59, 63

Index

Index